THE AUTHOR

Rosemary Conley is the UK's leading diet and fitness expert. Her diet and fitness books and videos have consistently topped the bestseller lists with combined sales in excess of nine million copies. Rosemary has also presented more than 300 cookery programmes on TV. In 2001 Rosemary was made an Honorary Freeman of the City of Leicester, and in 2004 she was awarded a CBE for services to the 'fitness and diet industries'.

Together with her husband, Mike Rimmington, Rosemary runs four companies: Rosemary Conley Diet and Fitness Clubs, which operates an award-winning national network of almost 200 franchises running over 2,000 classes weekly; Quorn House Publishing Ltd, which publishes *Rosemary Conley Diet & Fitness* magazine; Rosemary Conley Licences Ltd; and Rosemary Conley Enterprises.

Rosemary Conley's
Ultimate
Gi Jeans Diet

The healthiest and most effective
weight-loss plan – ever!

arrow books

Published in the United Kingdom by Arrow Books in 2007

1 3 5 7 9 10 8 6 4 2

Arrow Books
Random House Group Limited
20 Vauxhall Bridge Road, London SW1V 2SA

Addresses for companies within The Random House Group Limited can be found at: www.randomhouse.co.uk/offices.htm

The Random House Group Limited Reg. No. 954009

A CIP catalogue record for this book is available from the British Library

ISBN 9780099505594

The Random House Group Limited makes every effort to ensure that papers used in its books are made from trees that have been legally sourced from well-managed and credibly certified forests. Our paper procurement policy can be found at: www.randomhouse.co.uk/paper.htm

Edited by Jan Bowmer
Designed by Roger Walker

Typeset in Foundry Form Sans

Printed and bound in Great Britain by Bookmarque Ltd, Croydon, Surrey

Acknowledgments

It quickly became obvious that I should write a sequel to my original *Gi Jeans Diet* after so many people wrote to me with details of their astonishing success and the health benefits they enjoyed. This *Ultimate Gi Jeans Diet* represents a culmination of research and new ideas that greatly expands on the original diet, and I would like to thank Dr Susan Jebb, one of the UK's leading nutrition scientists, for her expert advice and guidance.

Thanks also to the team at ITV Central for giving me the opportunity to test the diet on television; to Teresa Keates for testing the Solo Slim Diet; to my husband, Mike, for testing the Kick-start Diet and for his encouragement throughout the writing of this book; to my daughter, Dawn, for her invaluable support, research and ideas in making this diet as extensive as possible.

I want to say a very big thank you to ALL the members who took the time to fill in the questionnaire; to our franchisees who gave out the forms and encouraged their members to complete them; and to our special team at Quorn House for inputting the information. I must also acknowledge the contribution made by Chris Ash, our Group Marketing Manager, and Angie Higgins, our General Manager, in compiling a questionnaire that is really useful and motivational; and to Jeremy Bromley, our IT manager, for creating a computer programme to collate the information.

A huge thank you, too, to my friend and colleague, Mary Morris, M.Sc., our Clubs' Training Consultant. Mary's expertise and knowledge forms the basis of all the exercise programmes in our magazine as well as in this and many other of my books. We also choreographed my new Gi Jeans Weight-loss Workout DVD together. Mary created the fascinating lifestyle quiz that appears in chapter 5 of this book, in consultation with Dr Susan Jebb. Mary is a total joy to work with and it is difficult to put into words how much I appreciate her.

I also want to thank Anne-Marie Littlewood, B.Sc., a former Clubs franchisee who is now Consultant for our online slimming club, rosemaryconleyonline.com. Anne-Marie sorted out the most commonly asked questions about low-Gi eating to help give readers a better understanding of how this diet works.

The recipes in this book are created by chef Dean Simpole-Clarke. Dean has a flair for producing easy-to-prepare, low-fat dishes that are suitable both for everyday eating and dinner parties. Thank you so much for all your skill and hard work, Dean.

All the meal suggestions and recipes are fat- and calorie-counted, and this extensive research was undertaken by my very patient PA, Melody Patterson. Thank you, Melody, for coping with this mammoth job alongside your other work.

Thanks must also go to everyone involved in turning my raw manuscript into this book: to Hannah Black at Century; to Roger Walker for designing the inside pages; to the cover design team; to hair and make-up artist Jane Tyler for making me look my best in the pictures; to Martin Black for the exercise photography; and to Allan Olley for taking such a great cover shot.

Last, but by no means least, thank you to my long-suffering book editor, Jan Bowmer. When I write a book, I don't have the luxury of time to go away for a month or so and work on it in one go. Anyway, this isn't that sort of book. There are so many different elements to it and it is only through Jan's expertise and patience that the book emerges as an understandable and hopefully inspiring volume! Thank you so much, Jan.

Useful information

Cooking weight conversions

Ounce (oz)	Pound (lb)	Gram (g)
1		25
2		50
3		75
4	¼	115
6		175
8	½	225
16	1	450
	1½	675
	2	1kg

Liquid measures

Fluid ounce (fl oz)	Pint	Millilitre (ml)
2		50
4		120
5	¼	150
6		175
8		250
10	½	300
12		350
14		400
	¾	450
16		475
	1	600
	1¼	750
	1½	900
	2	1.2 litres

Body weight conversions

Pound (lb)	Stone (st)	Kilogram (kg)	Pound (lb)	Stone (st)	Kilogram (kg)
1		0.5	9		4.1
2		1	10		4.5
3		1.4	11		5
4		1.8	12		5.4
5		2.3	13		5.9
6		2.7	14	1	6.3
7	½	3.2	28	2	12.7
8		3.6			

Spoon measures

1 teaspoon (tsp) = 5ml	1 tablespoon (tbsp) = 15ml

Linear measurements

Inch (in)	Feet (ft)	Millimetre (mm)	Centimetre (cm)
⅛		3	
¼		5	
½			2.5
1½			4
2			5
2½			6
3			7.5
3½			9
4			10
5			13
6			15
7			18
8			20
9			23
10			25
12	1		30

Abbreviations and symbols used

oz	ounce	ft	foot
lb	pound	mm	millimetre
g	gram	cm	centimetre
kg	kilogram	kcal	calorie
st	stone	tsp	teaspoon
fl oz	fluid ounce	tbsp	tablespoon
ml	millilitre	Ⓥ	suitable for vegetarians
in	inch	❄	suitable for home freezing

Contents

1 Lose weight fast!

I challenge you to find another diet that will enable you to lose weight faster or more healthily than this one! It's been tried and tested by thousands of dieters and really is the Ultimate Gi Jeans Diet! And because the eating plan is based on healthy and filling, low-fat, low-Gi foods, you won't feel hungry as the weight and inches drop away.

Since my *Gi Jeans Diet* book was published in January 2006, I have received thousands of letters and emails from readers telling me of their amazing successes on this revolutionary, easy-to-follow diet.

For instance, Angela McArthur from Glasgow wrote: 'I have lost 3st in 18 weeks and dropped from a dress size 18/20 to a size 12! People don't recognise me in the street and even my partner walked past me the other day! It has given me such a boost – I have more confidence, and I feel healthier and less tired.'

Sarah Bowyer, from Reading in Berkshire, lost 2st 6lb in eight weeks and wrote: 'I love this diet! The weight and the inches have dropped off me and I don't feel hungry. It's incredible!'

Adelle Smith, also from Reading, wrote: 'I have been on loads of diets over the years but never have I experienced the speed of weight loss like this. I have lost 6st in seven months. It's brilliant!'

Alison Hicks from Cheshire, who lost 1st 8½lb in eight weeks, wrote: 'My health and general wellbeing has improved beyond all expectations. Seeing the results so quickly has really encouraged me to stick with it.'

Carrie Masters, a diabetic from Surrey, also lost 1st 8½lb in eight weeks and wrote: 'The Gi Jeans Diet has worked brilliantly alongside my diabetes. I've never felt so well and have been able to reduce my insulin intake.'

I have been helping people to lose weight and get fitter for a long time and, with 27 diet books already under my belt, I thought I had written everything that I could to help overweight people become slimmer. But then I discovered the glycaemic index, or 'Gi' way of eating. Not only did it transform my own daily diet, but it inspired me to create my own Gi Jeans Diet and put it in a book. When it was introduced to Rosemary Conley Clubs around the UK the results were astonishing. Never, ever before had members experienced such enormous weight losses so fast.

So what exactly is Gi? Different foods cause our blood sugar levels to rise and fall at varying rates, immediately after we have eaten them and during the period following consumption. Foods with a low glycaemic index cause our blood sugar levels to rise slowly and fall gradually, which helps us to stay feeling full for longer. And this, of course, helps us when we are trying to lose weight. Avoiding sudden rises and falls in our blood glucose levels also is much better for our general health. Clinical research studies show that a low-Gi eating plan can reduce the risk of developing diabetes or heart disease. So many people these days are at risk of these diseases and a low-Gi diet is a real health-enhancer for all of us.

With this Ultimate Gi Jeans Diet, not only will you lose your unwanted weight safely and faster than ever, you will transform your shape and discover the body you have always wanted. Yes, really! Indeed, some research studies have shown that a low-Gi diet can maximise fat loss and in particular help reduce abdominal (tummy) fat.

This diet presses all the right buttons to allow you to achieve a fast but healthy weight loss yet offers sufficient food to satisfy the most demanding of appetites. Eating low-Gi foods prevents sudden food cravings, which are one of the main reasons dieters fail. In a moment of hunger they reach for that sweet or high-fat snack which then ruins the most effective of diets.

Unlike in many other Gi diets, all the foods included in this diet are also low in fat. Eating a low-fat diet minimises fat deposits around our bodies as, quite naturally, the fat we eat is stored as fat for emergencies in case we should ever find ourselves in the middle of a famine. As this is highly unlikely in the western world in the 21st century, we need much, much, less fat than we used to years ago when families had to 'make do' with whatever food was available.

Get the balance right

Losing weight is a matter of physics. Our bodies need fuel in exactly the same way as our cars need it. We eat food as fuel and, if we eat less than our bodies use up, we lose weight because the body has to get the fuel it needs from somewhere else. It does this by using some of its reserves from its existing fat stores. The opposite of this of course is if we eat more fuel than our bodies need, we gain weight, just like putting extra cans of fuel in our car boot. To keep our weight constant, we must eat an equal amount of food to what our bodies spend in energy. It's a fine balance.

The energy content of food is measured in calories and the trick is to select foods that we enjoy and which make us feel full but contain only a moderate number of calories. As I've done all the selecting and calculations for you in the menus in this book, there's no need for you to worry about calorie counting every item of food you eat. And as all the meal suggestions are based on low-fat foods, you will automatically be cutting down on lots of calories, anyway. Be aware that fat contains twice as many calories compared to other food groups. So, if we cut down the fat, we automatically cut down on the calories. Add to the mix some slow-energy-releasing, low-Gi foods and we naturally feel fuller for longer.

By eating in this way we don't feel hungry even though we are eating less fuel than the body uses. And, as the body demands a certain number of calories to fulfil its tasks and oper-ation, it automatically uses some of our stored fat to make up the difference. Then, if we include some extra activity, the body has to use even more fat from our fat stores to meet its extra needs. Result: fantastic weight and inch loss.

Get off to a flying start!

How this diet works is simple. To help get you off to a flying start I suggest that for the first two weeks you follow the Kick-start Diet. This strict but highly effective diet will enable you to lose around 7lb in 14 days. I can be confident in predicting this as in my initial trials with 36 volunteers, the average weight loss over two weeks was 7.25lb. Since that initial trial some dieters have even been known to lose up to a stone in two weeks but, of course, it all depends on how much weight you have to lose in the first place. What I do know is that I have never seen weight fall off people so fast and yet the diet is very healthy for adult men and women of all ages, irrespective of their starting weight.

After this initial two-week period, when you are asked to abstain from alcohol and treats, you should move on to Part 2 of the diet, which allows you more food choices. You will have more calories to play with, including an optional daily high-fat treat, plus a 100-calorie allowance for alcohol each day. The treats and the alcohol can be saved up over seven days if you wish so that you can still enjoy a very social weekend or special meal out.

You will be able to calculate your ideal personal calorie allowance by referring to the basal metabolic rate (BMR) tables at the back of this book. As you lose weight you will be able to adjust your calorie allowance accordingly so that you are always able to experience a significant weekly weight loss.

As I mentioned earlier, you do not have to get too involved in counting the calories in individual foods. I have included a wide selection of breakfast, lunch and dinner suggestions where all the calories have been carefully calculated. All you need to do is select meals within a calorie bracket, which, when totted up at the end of the day, do not exceed your total daily calorie allowance. This is fully explained later.

Unless otherwise stated in the diet plans, all foods contain five per cent or less fat – that's five grams or less fat per 100 grams of product. This will still give you a wide selection of foods to choose from but is a good rule of thumb to help steer you away from high-fat foods that will just make you fat! One important exception to this rule is oily fish, as it contains valuable nutrients. Health experts recommend eating at least one portion of oily fish every week.

Speed up your weight loss

At the same time as following the diet I recommend you increase your activity levels. This will not only increase the speed at which you lose weight but it will also help maximise your inch loss and help you to tone up as you slim down.

'Aerobic' exercise (that's activities such as walking, jogging, swimming and dancing) burns fat from our bodies, so it is a great way to speed up the weight-loss progress. Body toning exercises help strengthen our muscles, which makes them a better shape and also increases our ability to burn fat when we exercise aerobically.

Exercise is a good habit to get into, but sometimes our busy lifestyles prevent us from taking the time to do it and it slips down our list of priorities. It is really important that you develop the habit of becoming naturally more active. Treat yourself to a pedometer and wear it every day. It will greatly motivate you to think about moving more. Start by increasing your usual number of steps by an extra 2000 a day until you achieve 10,000 steps a day. Being more active will help you to become healthier, fitter and, of course, slimmer!

In chapter 3 I explain the principles of low Gi and advise how you can make some simple choices when selecting foods so that you can steer your day-to-day eating habits towards low-Gi foods. Not every food you eat needs to be low Gi, but introducing more low-Gi foods into your daily diet will benefit your health, too. Since I researched my original Gi Jeans Diet my husband, Mike, and I have switched effortlessly to eating low-Gi foods and we feel much better for it.

You have bought this book to help you transform your body and your health. I've been overweight myself, so I can empathise with you and I want to help you on your journey to a new you. If you follow the advice, stick rigidly to the diet principles and do some form of exercise or activity on at least five days a week, I guarantee you will succeed. Tens of thousands of Rosemary Conley Club members have proved without a shadow of a doubt that this diet works. If they can do it, so can you!

2 They did it, so can you!

At the same time as my original Gi Jeans Diet was launched in January 2006, ITV Central invited five brave folk to try the diet in the full glare of the television cameras. Sue Jinks, Sue Rea, Anne Hubbard, Jayne Marshall, and Tony Kemp, all from the Midlands, weighed in for everyone to see. With varying amounts of weight to lose, they took up the challenge with enthusiasm and sportsmanship. I kept in telephone contact with them and each time I phoned they were so positive and kept telling me how well they felt. It was really exciting.

Their second public weigh-in was after the initial two weeks on the Kick-start Diet, and the results sounded promising. Jayne had lost an impressive 8lb, Sue Jinks 7lb, little Sue Rea (as she became known because of her 5ft height) 7lb, Anne Hubbard 8lb, while our male dieter, Tony, had lost an impressive 1st 2lb in the fortnight and his trousers were nearly falling down!

The next weigh-in for the cameras was seven weeks later. We all met at Marks & Spencer at Fosse Park, a retail shopping centre on the outskirts of Leicester, so that we could get them all fitted out in new clothes for their now trimmer figures in time for the TV broadcast later that day. They all looked so much slimmer I couldn't have been more thrilled with their progress. After our shopping trip we went over to our offices at Quorn House where the TV cameras were ready for us. It was all very exciting.

The fab five were interviewed and then it was time for the final weigh-in. Ironically, on this particular day I had completely lost my voice, having had an attack of laryngitis over the previous few days. I couldn't utter a sound! I was so frustrated! However, Central News presenter Sameena Ali-Khan did a great job announcing the final weights, to the total shock, surprise and delight of the dieters.

After nine weeks Jayne had slimmed down from 11st 3lb to 9st 13lb – a loss of 1st 4lb. Sue Jinks had slimmed down from 12st 6lb to 10st 7lb – a loss of 1st 13lb! Little Sue Rea had shrunk from 10st 2lb to 9st 2lb – a stone lighter – while Anne Hubbard had slimmed from 12st 6lb to 11st 1lb – a loss of 1st 5lb. Then there was Tony. Tony had weighed in at 18st, which was far too much for his 5ft 10in frame, but in just nine weeks he lost an astonishing 2st 2lb and weighed in at a very reasonable 15st 12lb.

Tony, who lives in Nottingham, had been in denial about his weight until his trousers split. He said:

> 'I was so pleased to be selected for the TV trial. It was just what I needed and I couldn't believe how easy the diet was to follow. I didn't feel hungry and I felt so much better in myself. I know I will continue as it is just a way of eating now.'

When Tony and I met up again a few weeks later, he had lost another stone. Fabulous!

Anne Hubbard, from Leicestershire, found her weight had crept up over the years and size 16 clothes were getting tighter.

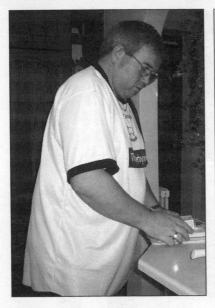

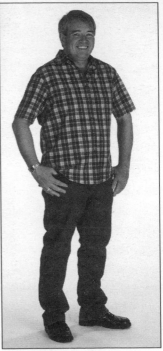

Tony Kemp at 18st

Tony lost 3st 2lb

After just nine weeks on the diet, Anne was wearing size 12 jeans! In that time Anne had lost 2in from her waist, 3in from her hips and 4in from her thighs. She said:

> 'I found the diet so easy to stick to and I enjoyed the recipes – as did the whole family, and I loved the exercise. I work out to Rosemary's *Shape Up & Salsacise* DVD four times a week as well as going to a class. I have so much more energy now.'

Anne also commented that she used to suffer with high blood pressure, but since losing her excess weight and exercising more her blood pressure was now normal. What's more she was now

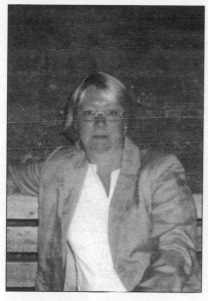

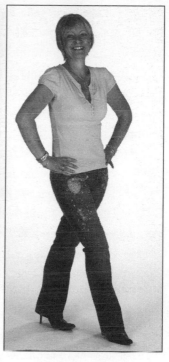

Anne Hubbard at 12st 6lb

Anne lost 3st

wearing size 10 trousers, which she hadn't done for 20 years!

I couldn't have wished for a more pleasant, happier bunch of people to try my diet and I know they still keep in touch with each other now.

In July, seven months after the TV trial started, Anne sent me a text message, which read: 'Just wanted to say thank you, have now lost 3st and just bought size eight jeans! Feel fantastic!'

When my original Gi Jeans Diet was launched in Rosemary Conley Diet and Fitness Club classes throughout the UK in 2006, we were all astonished at the fast and positive results achieved by members. Never before had we experienced weight losses like it and it wasn't long before our wonderful instructors were passing on to me the news of record-breaking rates of success. For instance, Lindsey Peters, a Hertfordshire franchisee, totted up her members' weight losses in January alone. They had lost over 100st in four weeks on the new diet!

News started spreading fast and new members were flocking to our classes and, as the *Gi Jeans Diet* had become a bestseller, my publishers were soon asking for a follow-up book. Having followed a similar pattern with my *Complete Hip and Thigh Diet* after the great success of my original *Hip and Thigh Diet* back in 1988, I thought it would be fun to write the *Ultimate Gi Jeans Diet*. As with my *Hip and Thigh Diet*, I also felt it would be interesting to carry out some further research into the actual statistical evidence produced by those who had followed this diet.

We created a questionnaire to be filled in only by those Rosemary Conley class members across the UK who had joined since my Gi Jeans Diet was launched in the Clubs – some four months previously. I wanted to compare their weight losses with those of members of the original trial team who had tested the diet through my local radio station, BBC Radio Leicester. In that original trial there were 36 willing volunteers who followed the diet for eight weeks. The results were extremely encouraging, with an average weight loss over the first two weeks of 7.25lb, and their average weight loss after eight weeks was an impressive 1st 1.5lb.

As the initial trial was done with a relatively small number of people, I was keen to see what the results might tell us if we cast the net further afield. So in May 2006 at the Rosemary Conley annual training convention at Center Parcs, our franchisees each took a few questionnaires to be completed by their members and returned by the end of July in time for me to finish this book. By mid-July I had received 382 questionnaires and these were analysed through a special computer programme designed by our IT manager, Jeremy. Members of staff input the data, then Jeremy pressed the button to print out the results. When I first saw that the average weight loss across 382 people was 1st 6lb in eight weeks I was flabbergasted. It seemed almost unbelievable but it was, of course, totally genuine. Yes, this diet really did work fast. Moreover, the dieters didn't find the diet difficult and spoke encouragingly of their successes. Here's a summary of the results.

The trial results

The trial participants covered a very wide age range. There were only four per cent in the 16–24 age group, 13 per cent in the 25–34 age bracket, 34 per cent in the 35–44 range, 27 per cent in the 45–54 age group, 15 per cent in the 55–64 range, and seven per cent were aged between 65 and 74.

The Kick-start Diet is tough and requires a couple of weeks of discipline and abstinence from alcohol, with the sole purpose of getting you off to a flying start to inspire you to continue. When asked 'Did you feel hungry on the Kick-start Diet?' 27 per cent said 'not at all', 31 per cent said 'hardly ever' while 38 per cent said 'occasionally'. Only four per cent said they were hungry 'very often'. I was surprised at how well they had coped.

When asked if they found the Kick-start Diet easy to follow, 51 per cent said it was 'very easy', 45 per cent said it was 'quite easy' while only three per cent said it was 'not easy' and one per cent said it was 'hard'.

But the results were astonishing and there is no doubt that, pushing ourselves hard when our motivation is at its highest and then seeing almost immediate results is immensely encouraging.

John Midgley, from Haworth in Yorkshire, lost 10½lb on the Kick-start Diet and went on to lose 3st 6½lb in 12 weeks. John commented that he also had given up smoking as well as joining the class and, along with the weight, almost all his symptoms of asthma had disappeared, too. His waist measurement went from 42in to 36in and he was delighted that his fitness level was 'better than ever!'

Wendy, from Devon, who lost 12lb in the first two weeks and went on to lose 3st 5lb in 16 weeks, also reported a considerable improvement in her asthma symptoms. She wrote:

'I'm amazed how easy it has been to lose the weight. Almost every day somebody tells me how amazing I look now – very good for my confidence.'

I was interested to find out how dieters had fared on my diet compared with other diets. One of the features of the Gi Jeans Diet is that it should make you feel full for longer than on other diets, so was this actually true? But I needn't have worried as 74 per cent said they were less hungry than on other diets while 13 per cent admitted to being slightly less hungry. Eleven per cent said they felt the same and only two per cent said they were more hungry.

Louisa Day from Hampshire wrote:

'I've found the diet easy to stick to and follow. I was never hungry and I have found my weight loss to be beneficial to my health. I am able to walk my dog further without losing my breath and it's boosted my self-confidence no end! Thank you.'

This diet is high in fibre-rich foods and not everyone can take to that, so I asked how dieters had coped. No one said they didn't like it, five per cent said they had coped, but 26 per cent said they didn't mind the high-fibre foods while the vast majority, 69 per cent, said they actually enjoyed it!

I went on to ask if the dieters felt they could continue eating this type of diet into the future. I was delighted to see that an overwhelming 79 per cent said 'certainly' and the remaining 21 per cent said 'probably'.

I then asked about overall health benefits and only one per cent said they didn't feel any different. A further eight per cent said they thought they felt healthier but an overwhelming 91 per cent said that they definitely did.

I was very pleasantly surprised at the many and varied health benefits that dieters reported. These included lowering of blood pressure and cholesterol, improved sleeping patterns, better skin, hair and nail condition, diabetes easier to control, big improvements in symptoms of irritable bowel syndrome (IBS) and polycystic ovary syndrome (PCOS), plus many more.

Here is a small selection of slimmers' comments on the health benefits they experienced.

Arthritis and joint problems

Alice Frape from Somerset wanted to lose weight because of her arthritic knees. Having followed the diet for 16 weeks and lost 2st 4lb, Alice wrote:

'My knees are easier and less painful and I feel my posture is better. I got myself a dog to increase my exercise level and my pace of my walking is steadily improving – thanks to the weight loss and the dog! I am enjoying the Gi Jeans Diet as it gives me so much freedom in what to eat. I have never worn jeans before I started this diet but am enjoying them now.'

Jenny Insley, from the Isle of Wight, commented:

'I have arthritis in my left knee. Since losing weight I can run up and down the stairs. I hardly have any pain at all now.'

Jean McAndrew, from Kilmarnock, wrote:

'Before I started the Gi Jeans Diet I had problems with my health; osteoarthritis in both knees, lower back problems and severe heel pain in both feet. So far the diet has improved my overall mobility and the weight loss [2st 4lb] has given me the determination to keep going so that I will feel even better when I reach my target weight. In the time that I have lost my first 2st my husband has lost 1½st. We both really enjoy the food we eat now as it tastes much better, we never feel hungry and we know exactly what we are eating. It is easily the best diet I have ever been on and it definitely makes you feel a lot healthier. When I reach my target weight I am determined NEVER to go back to my old way of eating.'

Shirley Harris from Bromsgrove wrote:

'It has definitely made a big difference to my joints and made me feel good about the way I feel and look. It is wonderful to hear my work colleagues making fun of me, saying I looked like a clown in my baggy trousers after only a few weeks.'

Carole Pardy from Oxfordshire wrote:

'I have had a problem with my knee and, with the combination of my 1st 6½lb weight loss and regular exercise, I have less pain and can walk miles!'

Asthma

Helen Rhodes from Kent wrote:

'My asthma has greatly improved, my skin has improved drastically as I always suffered from terrible acne. I can also run a lot further and enjoy exercising rather than dreading it. My sleep pattern has also greatly improved. I used to have disturbed sleep and minimal sleep but now I sleep right through the night and so have more energy.'

Blood pressure and cholesterol

Mrs D. J. from Wales wrote:

'I joined the class mainly because I had a cholesterol problem and if I couldn't get my weight down, tablets were the next option. I had a blood test three months after joining the class to find my blood pressure had reduced and there was no need for tablets.'

Julia Whittaker from Ashton-under-Lyne wrote:

'The reason for initially attending a Rosemary Conley class was due to being diagnosed with high cholesterol. This has reduced dramatically since undertaking this new diet and lifestyle change to what is now described as a "normal" level. Having been overweight for many years, I had forgotten just how much it impacts on your daily life. I now feel so much more confident in everyday situations, the health benefits are numerous and the fact that I can buy fashionable clothing from anywhere is just brilliant! This is my new lifestyle now and I never want to go back to being fat, frumpy and fed up!'

Jackie Petherbridge from Weston-super-Mare lost 2st 1lb since joining the class, which she feels has changed her life. She wrote:

'My six-monthly diabetic blood sample reading showed a dramatic decrease in cholesterol – my doctor was amazed. He thought I must be on statins! It is so easy to incorporate low-Gi foods into everyday eating and basic recipes. My cholesterol decrease is amazing.'

Sallie Watson from York lost 2st 5½lb in 13 weeks. She wrote:

'Extremely pleased with the results so far. Both my blood pressure and cholesterol have gone down. The Gi Jeans Diet doesn't seem like a diet – more of a lifestyle change.'

Helen Sherwin from Woking in Surrey lost 3st 3½lb in 16 weeks, and nearly a stone in the first two weeks. Helen told me:

> 'My goal when I started the Gi Jeans Diet in January was to go on holiday lighter than my husband and our two friends, as I have always been the heaviest by a long way. I achieved that the week we went away in May (over 3st lighter) and I was ecstatic! When I started this diet I had high blood pressure and raised cholesterol but my blood pressure is now normal and my cholesterol is lower.'

Breast cancer

Julie Sweetman from Hove lost 1st 11lb in 16 weeks. She wrote:

> 'At the beginning of last year I had an operation for breast cancer and subsequently have been taking Tamoxifen. My surgeon, at the time, told me that I would be wasting my money on joining a slimming club as I would not be able to lose weight on Tamoxifen. Thankfully, I am pleased to have proved him wrong.'

Diabetes

Lots of members wrote to me about the huge benefits to their diabetes. Here is a small sample of letters to encourage other diabetics who may be new to this diet.

Yvonne Harris from West Glamorgan wrote:

> 'I was diagnosed with Type 2 diabetes and have had very high blood pressure for 20 years. I have never

done much exercise and I joined other diet clubs, failing miserably. I joined my local Rosemary Conley class in January, then I attended my half yearly diabetic clinic in May and found to my amazement that everything was nearly normal, e.g. my cholesterol, blood pressure and sugar levels. The doctor even said that if I can manage to lose the same [1st 6lb] by the time I go back in November he would stop all my medication. Wow! How amazing is that and what a goal to aim for and stay with for a healthy, fitter life with bags of energy that I need for my 18-month-old grandson!'

Margaret York from Colchester lost 2st 1lb in 20 weeks. She wrote:

'This is the perfect combination for me – low fat and low Gi. I've never enjoyed exercise but I really love the classes. My diabetes nurse is very pleased with my results so far and I no longer feel myself becoming disabled. My blood sugars are way down and eating less fat also reduces the discomfort from my hernia, plus my feet and ankles are no longer swollen or painful.'

Jacqueline Gibson from Suffolk lost 1st 6½lb in 12 weeks. She wrote:

'I attended my diabetic clinic last week and the nurse was very pleased with me indeed. My blood pressure was right down to 108/63 and my sugar levels had dropped dramatically and were the lowest they have ever been, so the nurse printed off a graph for me. She said that she was going to keep my graph to show others how diet and exercise can reduce sugar levels. All this is due to attending the classes.'

Susan Taylor, one of my online slimmers, wrote:

'I've lost 6lb and my husband lost 7lb in the first week of the Kick-start Diet. In addition we have already seen major health benefits, particularly for my husband who is diabetic. His blood glucose levels were at 25–30 despite medication. Now, after just one week, they are at 8 and virtually within the normal range for a non-diabetic.'

Depression

Mrs T. D. from West Bromwich lost 2st 4½lb in 14 weeks and wrote:

'Although I still have nearly 3st to go to reach what I would like to weigh (9st), I have already gone from a size 22 to a size 16 on the Gi Jeans Diet. I have also recently squashed into a size 14 and I am determined to get to a size 10! So many people have commented on the weight loss and the general healthy glow I seem to have because I am losing the weight that has made me miserable for so long. I used to hate the sunshine and summer because I would have to endure hot weather in baggy tops and big coats to hide the fat, but now I recently have been out in jeans and a T-shirt! I used to puff and pant to get up the stairs, but now I carry a full washing basket up the stairs without putting it down or resting. The health benefits I have noticed most are my breathing, my circulation (I now have warm feet after having constantly cold feet), and less aching joints. Perhaps the most noticeable to me and everyone around me is the reduction in my feeling depressed. I will have a laugh now. Joining my local Rosemary Conley class is the best thing I have ever done. Everyone is friendly and in the same boat as I am. Thank you!'

Rachel Cox from Troon lost 2st 5½lb in 16 weeks and had suffered from postnatal depression. She wrote:

'I have found that losing the weight has improved my self-esteem. The "Gi" part of the diet has worked well at evening out my glucose levels that I was prone to. Also, this is the longest I have ever gone without gaining any weight – in my life! Four months and not a pound gained! Never has that happened before.'

Mrs G. H. from Hastings, who lost 12lb on the two-week Kick-start Diet and 3st 11lb after 19 weeks, wrote:

'Thank you for giving me my life back. I love the way I'm feeling right now. So much happier and fitter. My husband says I'm like a spring as I have so much energy. He thinks that I might explode as he has never seen me so happy!'

Heart problems

Maureen Whittles from Lytham wrote:

> 'I stopped smoking and put on 2st in weight. I needed a
> low-fat diet for cholesterol cut-down and your diet and
> exercise and my instructor Anne's smiling face cheering
> me on have made me in to an extremely fit person. I
> feet great.'

Headaches

Jayne Southall from Wolverhampton, who slimmed from 11st
11lb to 9st 12lb in 12 weeks, summed up so many of the comments made by others who completed questionnaires when she
wrote:

> 'I used to suffer regularly with headaches but since
> being on the Gi Jeans Diet I hardly suffer at all.'

Gastro-intestinal problems

Sue Brooks of Oxfordshire lost 2st 12½lb in 17 weeks and
reported:

> 'Everyone tells me I look ten years younger and I feel it!
> It is also great not to have the health problems that I
> had before. I had been referred to a colon specialist. By
> the time the appointment was confirmed I was on the
> diet and the symptoms had improved. He thought I was
> correcting the problem by my change of eating habits. I

had to go for a follow-up sigmoidoscopy, which was clear, and I now have no more problems. The diet has proved that a change in my eating has eliminated the problem.'

Premenstrual tension (PMT)

Mrs E. M. from Leeds lost 2st 4lb in 16 weeks and wrote:

'I am so much fitter. I can walk further in less time, I am less out of breath, less tired and more energetic. I am happy when I get out of bed each day. My PMT has reduced dramatically along with associated headaches, aches and pains.'

Sue Phillips from West Midlands lost 1st 11lb and wrote:

'I have lots of energy. My hair and skin, nails, etc. are great. I suffered badly from PMT – sore breasts, mood swings, hormonal spots, etc. – and these symptoms have disappeared.'

Sue went on to explain:

'I joined your classes with two friends – one has lost 3st 7lb and the other 1st 7lb. We walk, work out to a DVD in my shed every week and have a real laugh. As there are three of us it really motivates us and it means there are always at least two of us to exercise or go to class. We call ourselves "Fat Club" and are often the talk of the playground at school. We are really proud of what we have achieved.'

Underactive thyroid

Christine McCreadie from Swansea wrote:

> 'As I suffer from an underactive thyroid I find it very difficult to lose weight. I also had a hysterectomy six years ago and take HRT, which also does not help, so I am delighted with the results of your diet. After just eight weeks I have lost 1st 2lb.'

Gallstones

Sue Carter from Nottingham lost 2st on the diet and wrote:

> 'I feel generally healthier but also as I have gallstones the reduction of fat in my diet was very beneficial. It is a brilliant low-fat diet and I think one of the main factors for me has been the exercise at the class. This has encouraged me to do more exercise than I have ever done and it is the only diet that has REALLY changed my eating habits. A good instructor also makes a difference.'

Indigestion

Wendy Hollamby from Boston, who lost 9½lb on the Kick-start Diet and almost 2st after 12 weeks, wrote:

> 'Before I started the diet I used to suffer with terrible indigestion. It even used to wake me up during the night, but since starting the diet it has disappeared.'

Kim Hindle from Harpenden lost 1st 13lb in 16 weeks and wrote:

> 'I found that since eating wholegrain foods my abdomen feels a lot less bloated and so much more comfortable. My energy levels are much higher, which has improved my game of badminton, which I took up again on starting the diet. My indigestion has disappeared completely and my digestive system is no longer sluggish.'

Irritable bowel syndrome (IBS)

So many people remarked on a definite improvement in their IBS symptoms. Here are just a couple of comments.

Donna Hamillo from York lost 2st 10½lb in 16 weeks and wrote:

> 'I suffer from IBS, but since starting the diet and eating properly this has settled and I very rarely have an attack. I feel better than I have done in years and I have more energy and feel good about myself. I now have a regular eating pattern which I never had before.'

Sandra McIntyre, from Irvine in Scotland, lost 1st 13lb and wrote:

> 'Before starting the diet I had mild symptoms of IBS, but now I am eating more natural food and fibre I have no problems with this any more. My skin is a lot clearer and also brighter. Overall, I feel so much better.'

Menopause

Mrs J. B. from Tackley lost an impressive 3st 6½lb in 16 weeks and wrote:

'I am going through the menopause. I desperately wanted to lose the excess weight, as I know the increased dangers of contracting breast cancer (which my mother died of four years ago). My hot flushes and other unpleasant symptoms have practically disappeared and everyone – especially my husband – says I look ten years younger and gorgeous!'

Polycystic ovary syndrome (PCOS)

Jillian Liptrot from Wigan lost 2st 3lb in 10 weeks and attached a letter to her questionnaire. She wrote:

'Over the last three years I have suffered two still births due to a weak cervix. After losing the second baby I was referred to a specialist at Liverpool Women's Hospital where they did a number of tests. They found the cause of my weakness was the neck of the cervix and hopefully there is an operation to cure this. The only problem was that I had put on a lot of weight that needed to come off before my consultant was happy to do the operation.

'Having polycystic ovaries (PCO) means it's harder for me than most to lose weight. So I set off on a mission to try and lose weight so I could have the operation. First I tried to do it myself but no joy. I tried

Weight Watchers with no joy, then Slimming World again with no joy. I felt it was going to be impossible to do. Then one day I went to the supermarket and saw an advertisement for Rosemary Conley classes. I thought I haven't tried that one, so I popped in and the instructor went through the diet with me. Now I have lost 2st 3lb in just 10 weeks and – wait for it – I've been booked in to have my operation on 27 June and after that we will be able to start to try for a baby. Without your classes I don't know how long it would have taken me. I had some blood tests back in January because of my PCO and my hormone level was 4.1. At the beginning of May it was down to 2.8. My periods were very irregular but since losing weight they have become more regular.'

Cath Mulcahy from St Helens in Merseyside lost an astonishing 4st 12lb and wrote:

'I joined a Rosemary Conley class because I was told I had polycystic ovaries and that losing weight would help my symptoms and my health. Since losing weight and maintaining it I am completely symptom free. The effect of losing my weight has been unreal. The consultants at the hospital are all astonished.'

Body shape

I was interested to know which parts of the body most people wanted to slim down. This was a multiple choice question, so dieters could tick more than one box. Seventy-seven per cent said they wanted to lose weight from their stomach and 60 per cent off their waist. Hips attracted 68 per cent, with thighs scoring 58 per cent. Only 34 per cent wanted to lose weight off their bust, 32 per cent from their arms, and 13 per cent wanted to slim down their knees.

When I asked which part of their body had reduced significantly, the waist came out top at 48.5 per cent, followed by hips at 40 per cent, stomach at 38 per cent, thighs at 26 per cent and bust at 27 per cent. Knees and arms scored five per cent and six-and-a-half per cent respectively.

The excellent news is that these results indicate a loss of body fat, and as fat around the waist presents the most danger to the heart, to lose most fat from there has very significant health benefits.

Mrs A. N. from Swansea lost 1st 6lb in 17 weeks and wrote:

'My waist is down from 47in to 39in in 17 weeks. What I say to that is "Wow!"'

Linda Murphy from York wrote:

'My shape has altered amazingly and I need a whole new wardrobe. I have kept my biggest pair of trousers and try them on from time to time to confirm to myself just how much weight I have lost. My skin is much clearer and I am looking younger. I hated exercise at school and have always avoided it where possible – I love it now and feel terrible if I miss my regular exercise for some reason.'

Cellulite

For those who suffer with cellulite I asked the question 'Do you think your cellulite has reduced since following this diet?' While 51 per cent didn't know and just 10 per cent said it hadn't, 39 per cent felt that it definitely had. As only the pear-shaped dieters were likely to have cellulite anyway, I felt this was a very gratifying result.

Exercise

Next, I wanted to know how active everyone had been and I have to congratulate my trial team for showing such dedication to getting fitter. The question read: 'How often did you manage to do 20–30 minutes of some form of aerobic exercise?' Three per cent did no exercise at all and 20 per cent worked out once or twice a week. The majority, 40 per cent, managed three or four times a week, which is great, while 20 per cent achieved five workouts a week and 27 per cent managed to do something every day! Not surprisingly 97 per cent said the exercise had made a difference to their fitness levels and 89 per cent stated that it had definitely made a difference to their shape.

I was interested to know whether there was a change in attitude towards fitness as a result of the increased activity of the trialists and, indeed, 93 per cent said they had enjoyed exercising more since following the Gi Jeans Diet programme.

Pauline Beal from Scunthorpe lost 1st 4½lb in eight weeks. She wrote:

'I have always hated any form of exercise but since I have started the Gi Jeans Diet I have become a "born again" exerciser! I go to exercise classes three times a week and take long walks on the other two weekdays AND I ENJOY IT!'

Cheryl Ritchie from Kettering wrote:

'My energy levels have increased to the point that I cannot remember having felt so energetic before in my life. I find that I actually ENJOYED the exercise.'

Kate Hurley from West Sussex, who lost 1st 3lb in nine weeks, wrote:

'I have "discovered" exercise through salsacise and class exercise. It is great fun. My bad back has just about gone and I spring out of bed every morning!'

Dieting history

It is always interesting to understand dieters' history when putting statistical information together, so I enquired of my trial team. Not surprisingly, 44 per cent had been on more diets than they cared to remember, while 43 per cent acknowledged that they had only dieted occasionally, and 13 per cent said this was their first ever attempt at dieting.

Next I wanted to know whether the diehard dieters had found the Gi Jeans Diet more successful than other diets they had attempted. A massive 85 per cent indeed said that they found this diet more successful than others.

Then I asked a multi-choice question to find out which aspect of the diet they liked best so that I could bear this in mind when compiling future diets. The results read as follows:

It was easy to follow	64%
I didn't feel like it was a diet	53%
I didn't feel hungry on the diet	51%
It was good to be able to have a treat	46%
It offered more freedom of choice	45.5%
The Power Snacks helped me not to cheat	45%
I liked the food suggested	44.75%
I could have a drink and not feel guilty	34.5%
Counting the calories for each meal was easier than doing so for individual foods	34%
I could eat so much more than on most diets	26.5%

So, that was what the statistics told me and the comments from the trialists themselves were so encouraging. To finish this chapter here is a selection of general comments that I hope might encourage you to have a good shot at creating a new you!

Mrs J. P. from Weston-super-Mare lost 2st in 12 weeks and noticed ongoing improvements in her energy and fitness levels. She wrote:

'Mental alertness has improved and friends say I am radiating a healthy aura. My GP has recorded "Rosemary Conley Diet – very successful!" on my notes.'

Karen Morris from Nottingham, who lost 1st 7½lb in eight weeks and 2st by the time she sent in her questionnaire, wrote:

'My health is so much better. On the days I exercise I sleep so much better. I feel healthier and fitter and I have more energy. I feel wonderful, exhilarated. I feel on such a high, my self-esteem has risen, and I'm wearing new and fashionable clothes. I am a new woman! I thought I had lost these things for ever before I started the diet.'

Mrs M. M. from West Sussex wrote:

'I am amazed that I have now lost almost a stone without feeling hungry. At 63 years old I have found it almost impossible to lose the extra stone that was making me feel unattractive, lethargic and unfit. I am delighted with the results.'

Dawn Akerman from Berkshire wrote:

'I am 40 this year and wanted to be fab and fit at 40. I think I've achieved this and I am certainly more active. My confidence has been given a big boost as people say how good I look. I have felt like a different person since being on the diet. I used to come home from work and fall asleep on the sofa. Not any more. I have more energy and generally feel a lot fitter. I have had thyroid cancer and put on a lot of weight after the operation. I got very depressed as well. Now I have lost nearly 1½st, I feel so much better, my clothes fit and I have dropped a dress size. I was bordering on a size 14 but now I am a comfortable 10.'

Céean Morrison from Birmingham lost 1st 7lb in nine weeks and wrote:

'This Gi Jeans Diet does not feel like a diet at all. I am in love with this new life I have found. I have not felt tired any more, I have a lot more energy, my skin looks better and my hair is much healthier. I had two operations and after my illness this programme has given me a new start to my life and an amazing confidence boost! I can't believe how far I have come.'

Eileen McGuffie from Troon lost a remarkable 3st 4½lb in 17 weeks and wrote:

'I've lost the weight of my five-year-old daughter and I can't imagine how I managed to walk about carrying her weight all day!'

Amanda Houghton from Lincolnshire lost 2st 1½ lb in 19 weeks and wrote:

'I wake up each morning much brighter and alert. An added bonus is that my husband has lost 2st as well. Also my body fat percentage has come down from 43 per cent to 31 per cent. I've kept a diet and fitness journal and found that this has made me more aware of what I eat and drink. It has helped me cut down on my drinking and I don't miss that either!'

Joanna Sweet from Bolton lost 1st 10lb in 15 weeks. She wrote:

'My skin feels cleaner, and in general I have felt a lot more alert and ready to do things, especially in the afternoon. I was able to complete a 40-mile walk without feeling too tired afterwards!'

Ann Jones from Northampton didn't have a lot of weight to lose but lost her 1st 2lb in 12 weeks and remarked:

'The diet has taught me how to put less fat into my body, given me an incentive to exercise and made me a lot happier knowing I can get into size 10 jeans! I have never dieted properly before as I have no willpower but I have really enjoyed the exercise classes and have learned a lot. The discipline of the regular weigh-in and the class really made me focus on what I was putting into my body and how I was cooking it.'

And finally, Lorna O'Brien from Ayr in Scotland, who slimmed down from 12st 9½lb to 9st in 16 weeks, wrote:

'This is the best diet I've been on. It doesn't feel like a diet. I used to binge on massive amounts of chocolate, cakes and sweets and I don't have any cravings for these foods any more. I feel 100 times fitter and healthier. It's been so easy to follow and the recipes are great. It's helped having a fantastic instructor to keep me motivated and looking forward to each week with plenty of help and advice.'

Lorna lost 1st 3lb in the first eight weeks, 2st 11½lb after 12 weeks and a remarkable 3st 9½lb after 16 weeks. Lorna's figure shrank from a 41–35–41½in to a slimline 35–28–35in! What a transformation!

3 Gi made easy

Quite simply, the glycaemic index (Gi) is a way of ranking carbo-hydrate foods based on the rate at which they raise our blood sugar (glucose) levels. Carbohydrates are foods such as bread, rice, pasta, cereal and potatoes, although carbohydrate is also found in all fruits and vegetables and some other foods. The rate at which the energy from carbohydrate enters the bloodstream depends on many different factors, including the exact type of starch and the method of cooking.

Each food is given a rating and the lower the rating, the better. A rating above 70 is considered 'high' Gi, a rating between 69 to 55 'medium', and under 55 'low'. Most of the foods included in my Ultimate Gi Jeans Diet eating plan are low Gi but you can 'shift' the Gi value by combining different foods. So occasionally I have combined a 'high' Gi food with a 'low' Gi one to make a 'medium' Gi meal, which is still healthy.

Low-Gi diets are based largely around fibre-rich foods and include lots of fresh fruit and vegetables and generous helpings of legumes (beans and pulses). Fibre is a crucial component of any healthy low-Gi diet, and in many cases the higher the fibre content, the lower the Gi ranking is likely to be.

Gi and weight loss

Although studies have shown that eating low-Gi foods can help prevent certain health problems, no clinical trials have proved that a low-Gi diet on its own helps you to lose weight. That's not really surprising because we have known for a very long time that to lose weight we need to eat fewer calories than we actually use up each day. We also know that eating low-fat foods is an easy way to cut back on the calories as, compared with carbohydrates or proteins, gram for gram, fat contains twice as many calories. And, if we add into the mix some regular moderate exercise, we can speed up the weight-loss process as well as further improving our overall health and fitness.

A low-Gi diet therefore will only help weight loss if it helps to cut the calories. Low-Gi foods such as beans and pulses, fruit and vegetables are naturally low in calories. In addition the high fibre content of many low-Gi foods helps us to feel fuller for longer as the stomach doesn't empty as fast as it does after eating highly processed foods.

Be aware, though, that some low-Gi foods, such as peanuts, are high in fat, so the key is to choose low-fat foods, then select low-Gi ones, too. Remember, fat makes you fat! The most effective way to lose weight is to follow a low-fat, calorie-controlled diet and that is the difference between the diet in this book and many other Gi diets that have been published.

It is also important to realise that for the purposes of this weight-loss plan NOT EVERY food you eat needs to be low Gi. The aim is to eat a balanced, healthy diet that contains a high proportion of foods with a low or medium Gi rating and to choose healthy, low-fat options.

Glycaemic load

Glycaemic load (GL) is a calculation of the Gi value and carbohydrate content per serving of food. It takes into account the amount of carbohydrate in the meal and the type of carbohydrate (its Gi value). Both are equally important and they both have an effect on blood sugar levels. However, by incorporating low-Gi foods into your diet you will automatically reduce the glycaemic load.

The A–Z of Gi

A APPLES Whole apples and apple juice are low-Gi foods as half the sugar is fructose, which has a very low Gi rating.

B BANANAS These provide valuable energy. Choose slightly under-ripe ones for a lower Gi rating. Avoid over-ripe ones as they have a higher Gi.

C CEREALS Whole-oat or high-fibre breakfast cereals such as porridge, All-Bran, Bran Buds and Shredded Wheat are low-Gi foods. Special K is also a good choice. Weetabix is borderline medium Gi but is included in the diet plan because it is a natural low-fat, low-sugar option. See also MUESLI and OATS.

D DRIED APRICOTS These have a low Gi ranking but are high in calories – so try to avoid them while you are trying to lose weight!

E EGGS Because they contain minimal carbohydrate, eggs are zero-rated in Gi terms. The white of the egg is fat-free, but the yolk is high in fat, which is why you are restricted to two or three a week on my low-fat diets.

F FRUCTOSE Otherwise known as 'fruit sugar', fructose is found in all fruits as well as in honey. It is slowly absorbed into the bloodstream and does not stimulate the production of insulin. It has a low Gi ranking, but it does have the same number of calories as sucrose or 'table sugar'.

G GRAPEFRUIT While the whole fruit has a very low Gi ranking, grapefruit juice is much higher, so always go for the whole fruit, if you can.

H HERBS Fresh herbs can be used to enhance a variety of dishes to add flavour and interest, which is particularly important when preparing low-fat dishes. As well as being low Gi, they cut down on the need for salt and many contain other useful nutrients.

I ICE CREAM This has a medium-to-low Gi ranking, depending on the ingredients. As long as you count the calories, it can be included in a low-Gi eating plan.

J JASMINE RICE Avoid jasmine rice as it has the highest Gi ranking of all types of rice.

K KIDNEY BEANS Red kidney beans and other common bean varieties are a valuable low-Gi source of protein and fibre in any healthy eating plan. If you are adding kidney beans to a casserole, make sure they have been boiled for at least 10 minutes first.

L LENTILS With a very low Gi ranking and low calorie count, lentils are a valuable ingredient in any diet. While they taste quite bland in themselves, you can add flavour by cooking them in stock or adding herbs and other flavourings, and they are great for thickening soups and casseroles. Lentils are rich in protein, so they are ideal for vegetarians, and they also contain B vitamins and fibre.

M MUESLI It is the raw oats that help give this worthy cereal a low Gi ranking, because they take longer to digest. Weigh out your serving if you are counting calories, as you may fool yourself about your portion size, which could hinder your weight-loss efforts.

N NEW POTATOES Go for the waxy ones in their skins, as these have a lower Gi ranking than old potatoes.

O OATS are a highly nutritious low-Gi cereal. Make into porridge with water and serve with skimmed or semi-skimmed milk and a little fruit for a wholesome breakfast that will see you through the morning.

P PASTA A low-Gi food and perfect for the dieter – as long as you stick to tomato-based sauces instead of creamy ones.

Q QUARK This soft cheese is made from skimmed milk. Its low-fat, low-Gi properties makes it ideal for slimmers and it can be used instead of cream cheese in many recipes or to cream potatoes.

R RICE Basmati rice is the best low-Gi choice as it contains a type of starch called amylose, which gives it the lowest Gi rating of all common types of rice.

S SWEET POTATO This has the lowest Gi ranking of all potatoes and is versatile and deliciously different. Dry-roast, boil, or steam, and serve whole or mashed. You can even bake sweet potatoes in their skins and serve as jacket potatoes. Cook them in just the same way as ordinary old potatoes, but for a shorter time. Children love them, too.

T TORTELLINI This is small, crescent-shaped pasta that can be filled with a variety of foods from meat to cheese. Like all pasta, it is low Gi, but if you want to lose weight, stick to low-fat fillings.

U UNREFINED CARBOHYDRATES These contain more fibre and have a lower Gi rating than more refined varieties.

V VINEGAR Add vinegar to salads in place of oil. The acidity of vinegar slows digestion, which lowers the overall Gi rating of the meal.

W WHOLEGRAIN BREAD Select bread that has been made from stoneground or wholegrain flour. Or try pitta breads for a change, as these have a lower Gi than ordinary loaves.

X EXTRA VEGETABLES Fill up on plenty of these with your main meal. You can eat most vegetables without being too worried about their Gi ranking – or their calorie content – as long as you don't add butter or oil when cooking or serving them.

Y **YOGURT** is a real friend of the Gi dieter. The acidity and high protein content slow down the emptying of the stomach, plus it is rich in calcium. Choose low-fat varieties as these have fewer calories than high-fat ones. Rather than buying fruit yogurt, it is best to buy natural yogurt, and add your own fruit as fruit yogurts tend to have lots of added sugar.

Z **ZEST** This is the outer rind of citrus fruit that can be removed with a peeler or zester. It is used to add flavour to sweet or sour dishes or as a decoration or garnish.

A QUICK GUIDE TO LOW GI

- Choose whole-oat cereals for breakfast rather than refined corn or rice ones.
- Select wholegrain, multigrain or stoneground bread or loaves containing intact seeds and grains in place of ordinary white or brown bread.
- Pitta bread and tortilla wraps make great sandwich alternatives.
- Basmati rice has a lower Gi than other varieties of rice.
- Choose sweet potatoes or waxy, new potatoes cooked in their skins as these have a lower Gi than old potatoes.
- Pasta has a lower Gi than potatoes or rice.
- Add beans and pulses to stews and casseroles, salads and soups to reduce the overall Gi rating of your meal.
- Use low-calorie, low-Gi fillers such as tomatoes, beansprouts, chopped celery and courgettes to 'bulk up' meals and give you more chewing power.
- Avoid over-ripe bananas – they have a higher Gi than less ripe ones.
- Eat fruit in place of cakes and biscuits.

4 Your good health

In order for our bodies to function at their optimum level, we need to feed them a variety of essential nutrients. Nutrition doesn't have to be complicated; we just need to understand the five basic categories that nutrients fall into – protein, carbohydrate, vitamins, minerals, and fat.

We need protein for growth and repair, carbohydrates for energy, vitamins and minerals to boost our immune system and help cells and organs do their job. Lastly, we need some fat, also for energy.

Protein

Protein is vital for growth and repair of our body tissues. It is found in foods such as meat, fish, eggs, cheese and milk, and in non-animal sources, such as soya beans. Protein is very satiating and also helps you feel fuller for longer, so try to have a portion at each meal.

When following a low-fat diet it is also important to select protein foods carefully as some can be quite high in fat. Always go for lean cuts of meat, remove the skin from poultry, choose low-fat cheeses and skimmed or semi-skimmed milk in preference to full fat. Choosing low-fat versions of these foods does not in any way reduce the protein content but it does reduce the number of calories dramatically and will also benefit your heart. Oily fish falls into a category of its own, since the health benefits from the essential fatty acids it contains override its high fat content. Aim to eat at least one portion a week of oily fish such as mackerel, herring, or salmon.

Carbohydrates

Carbohydrates are vital for energy and can give us a sense of fullness after eating them. As carbohydrates are very easily burned by the body, they are not readily stored as body fat. Carbohydrate foods include bread, potatoes, rice, pasta and cereals.

On my Ultimate Gi Jeans Diet I recommend you consume some carbohydrate with every meal. Choose natural sources where possible and follow the Gi guidelines in chapter 3. Choose bread made with wholegrain or stoneground flour; select sweet potatoes or new potatoes with their skins on for extra fibre; all pasta is good but try to avoid high-fat sauces; opt for basmati rice in preference to other types; and choose high-fibre or oat-based breakfast cereals wherever possible.

Vitamins and minerals

Vitamins are important nutrients which occur naturally in food and form part of the family of micronutrients. These are nutrients that are essential for good health but only needed in very small (micro) amounts. Other micronutrients are minerals, such as iron and calcium, or trace elements, such as iodine or silicon, which are needed in minute (trace) amounts in the body.

There are many different kinds of vitamins, but they fall into two groups according to their chemical structure. Some, such as the group of B vitamins or vitamin C, are water-soluble. As the name suggests, these vitamins dissolve in water and are excreted from the body in urine. It is important to eat some of these nutrients every day. Others, such as vitamins A, D, E and K, are fat-soluble and are more easily stored by the body, so you can balance out your nutrient needs over a few days.

There is no single food that is essential, but choosing a varied and balanced diet will help you to obtain all the vitamins you need.

Vitamin A

This is a group of vitamins and it includes beta-carotene, which can be converted in the body to vitamin A. Vitamin A is essential for the immune system, for skin health and for good eyesight, especially in dim light. Carrots are rich in beta-carotene, which helps explain the old wives' tale that carrots help you see in the dark! Vitamin A is found in meat, especially liver, and oily fish, eggs and dairy produce. Beta-carotene occurs in yellow, orange and dark green fruit and vegetables such as mangoes, peppers, carrots and spinach.

There are some concerns that too much vitamin A may not be good for health. Large quantities during pregnancy can increase the risk of fetal abnormalities, and high intakes over many years may increase the risk of bone fractures in later life. Vitamin A is an antioxidant and it has been suggested that it may help reduce the risk of cancer. However, a study among smokers actually showed an increased risk of cancer in those taking vitamin A supplements.

If you eat liver or liver products such as pâté once a week you are likely to be eating the recommended amount of vitamin A and it may be advisable not to eat liver more often and to avoid supplements containing vitamin A. The Department of Health in the UK recommends you avoid eating liver while pregnant because of the specific risks to the unborn baby. There is no need to limit your intake of fruits and vegetables rich in beta-carotene.

Vitamin B

This is a whole family of vitamins with a range of different functions. B vitamins help to make red blood cells, which carry oxygen around the body and also metabolise food to produce energy. B vitamins are found in a wide variety of foods, including cereals, meat and dairy products.

The B vitamin folic acid is found in many vegetables and fruits and may be added to some other foods, such as breakfast cereals. Women who are planning a pregnancy or who are in the first 12 weeks of pregnancy should take a folic acid supplement (400 micrograms per day) to reduce the risk of having a baby with spina bifida.

Vitamin C

This is one of the best-known vitamins and over the years has been credited with curing everything from the common cold to cancer. Vitamin C is found in a wide variety of fruit and vegetables. Levels of vitamin C decrease while food is being stored, and vitamin C is easily destroyed by cooking. Choose very fresh or frozen fruit and vegetables and eat raw where possible, or cook only lightly, ideally steaming them or cooking in the microwave.

Vitamin C is essential for every cell in the body, including skin, blood vessels and even bones. It is a powerful antioxidant and helps the body to fight infections. It also helps the body to absorb iron efficiently from the gut into the bloodstream. However, there is little evidence that more than the recommended 40 milligrams of vitamin C a day – equivalent to a medium glass of orange juice – has any extra health benefits. Higher doses of vitamin C are simply excreted in urine, but a gram or more a day can cause diarrhoea.

Vitamin D

This is a curious vitamin, because in theory the body can make all the vitamin D it needs by the action of sunlight on the skin. Vitamin D is essential for healthy bones, and low intakes can lead to rickets in children or osteomalacia (a bone disease) in older people. Vitamin D is found in dairy foods, egg yolks, fatty fish and fish with small edible bones, such as sardines. Some foods, such as margarine, are fortified with vitamin D. Liver is a good source of vitamin D, but it is best not to consume this more than once a week because it contains high levels of vitamin A.

Most people can get all the vitamin D they need from their diet or the sunshine, but research shows that some groups of people may be at risk of vitamin D deficiency. The Department of Health in the UK recommends that pregnant or lactating women and older people who are most at risk of deficiency, could usefully take a vitamin D supplement of 10 micrograms a day. If you spend little time outdoors, apply lots of sun cream or are of Asian origin, you may also benefit from a similar supplement.

Vitamin E

Vitamin E is best known as an antioxidant which helps protect the cells of the body from damage. It is found in vegetable oils, wholegrains, nuts and seeds.

Vitamin K

This is one of the lesser-known nutrients. It is essential for efficient blood clotting, and new research suggests it is vital for good bone health, too. Vitamin K is found in green vegetables and in some vegetable oils. It is also produced by some bacteria in the gut.

Do you need a vitamin supplement?

National surveys in the UK show that most people eat the recommended quantities of vitamins and do not require extra supplements. However, as an insurance policy, especially if you are dieting, you may wish to take a general multi-vitamin supplement. Choose a product with a wide range of vitamins, rather than single nutrients. Check the label to choose one that provides about the recommended intake of the different vitamins.

Consider taking a multi-vitamin supplement if:

- You are dieting
- You have a poor appetite
- You have erratic eating habits
- You are a fussy or picky eater
- You eat less than five portions of fruit and vegetables a day.

Many people take fish oil supplements and these frequently include some of the fat-soluble vitamins. If you take more than one supplement, remember to add up the total amount of vitamin present. If you are pregnant, or have any medical condition, consult your doctor before taking any supplements as they may interfere with your condition or with other medications.

It is important to consume sufficient vitamins, but more is not better, and in some cases may even be harmful. Research repeatedly shows that people who eat a varied diet with plenty of fruit and vegetables tend to live longer, healthier lives, but there is no evidence that the same is true for supplement users. Remember that pills are a supplement – not a substitute – for a healthy diet.

Fat

While fat is important as part of a balanced healthy diet, these days we need very little to have enough. Centuries ago when supermarkets were not open 24/7 and we didn't drive cars, the human race survived because of foods from crops and animals. Every scrap was eaten, including all the fat from the animals, and the body was designed to store concentrated energy from fat as body fat for when there was little or no grain left and the meat was running out. This body fat then provided the necessary energy to keep people alive with what little grain or meat was left until the next harvest or until the animals reproduced.

Now that life is so different, we do not need anywhere near as much fat, yet high-fat food is all around us – in vending machines, petrol stations, restaurants and supermarkets – ready to tempt us. Not only are we eating more fat but, unfortunately, we are also burning fewer calories because our lives are not as physically demanding as they were in years gone by. It's no wonder that people are getting fatter.

As far as weight loss is concerned, it doesn't matter whether fat is saturated or polyunsaturated, it will still be stored as fat on your body. If you are suffering from heart disease, it is especially important to cut down on saturated fat. Your heart condition should also improve and even more so if you lose weight and take regular exercise. So, my simple advice to you is to eat low fat as a matter of course by selecting foods (except oily fish) that have five per cent or less fat. Do this, and you won't go short or be missing out on essential nutrients from fat. Remember, you cannot eat too little fat, as many foods, such as bread, cannot even be produced without using some fat.

I have been eating low-fat foods for 20 years and I have never felt better. My regular health checks, which include blood testing, confirm that everything is in very good order, so I am speaking from personal experience as well as under the guidance of nutritional experts.

And if you think that eating low fat might adversely affect your skin, nails or hair, it won't. So many of our trialists commented on how these had improved, without our even asking them the question.

For instance, Debbie Elton from Essex followed the diet with her daughter Amy. Debbie wrote:

'Overall, my health has improved considerably, there has been an improvement in my skin, the growth of my hair and nails plus I have gained lots of confidence.'

Mrs C. W., also from Essex, wrote:

> 'My fingernails always used to be splitting; now they get long enough for me to have to file them. I don't have to hide my hands now.'

Jo Keddie from Kent, who lost 2st 6½lb in 12 weeks, wrote:

> 'My skin is so much clearer, I no longer have any little aches and pains in my knees and lower back. I have more energy, and my confidence is so much better. I am generally a lot happier and I really like receiving compliments! I just feel better overall. This diet feels like one I could live with.'

Jane Murray from Berkshire commented:

> 'I have noticed that my general health, including nails, hair and skin, has improved. I feel more energetic and lively and I can now share my teenage daughter's clothes!'

5 How old are you *really*?

Looking younger than we really are is something most of us would like to achieve. For someone who looks older than their biological age, the tell-tale signs are often the condition of the skin on face and hands, a thickening of the waist and a change in posture. The reverse is also true, in that someone who looks younger than their biological age may have a clear and glowing skin and a good body shape and posture.

Take my mother-in-law, Jeanne, who is amazing and a total inspiration to us all. At 84 years young, she lives alone (her husband died six years ago), keeps her not-small house spotless, does all the gardening, makes her own bread, soups, yogurt, birthday cards, grows her own bedding plants and makes her own clothes! She always looks elegant – to the point that people stop her in shops or in the street and tell her so! Does Jeanne look her age? Not a bit of it. She is slim, walks well, keeps fit by staying active and keeps mentally alert by doing crosswords. Jeanne enjoys every single day and when I visit on most Saturdays, she cooks me a delicious lunch and is always bright and cheerful. I look forward to my visits.

Wouldn't we all like to be able to live such an independent life when we reach our 80s? The trouble is, real ageing goes a lot deeper than skin deep. How we live our life in terms of levels of stress and relaxation, drinking and eating, sleeping and exercise has a huge impact on our bodies, and many of us may be blissfully unaware of the effect until it is too late.

If leading an unhealthy lifestyle gave you large red blotches all over your face you would probably be motivated to do something about it. But, in reality, when the body is beginning to go wrong from the inside, as in the early stages of heart disease for example, there may be no sign at all of anything wrong, so most people think they are getting away with it. Most first heart attacks are fatal and in many cases there is real shock that it has happened despite everyone knowing that an unhealthy lifestyle may have been to blame. Adopting a healthy lifestyle is like taking out the best insurance policy you can buy. Making a few key lifestyle changes and sticking to them is all that is required to reverse the effects of ill health and enjoy the enormous benefits of looking and feeling healthier – and a lot younger!

The simple questionnaire that follows will be very revealing for you. It is based on your current lifestyle and will give you a score related to your lifestyle habits. A bad habit, such as smoking, gives you a high 'plus' score because we know that it can add years well beyond your real age. Your birth certificate may say you are only 43 but your body is functioning as if it were 63! By contrast, if you are a regular exerciser you can give yourself a 'minus' score as we know that people who exercise regularly are likely to take years off their real age and look and feel great!

This is not a scientific analysis and it is not meant to be. You would need to have some very specific tests taken by a medical practitioner to achieve that, but even this fun questionnaire can be a very good health indicator and may be the motivation you need to make those lifestyle changes.

Lifestyle questionnaire

To work out your *lifestyle* age compared to your *real* age, tick the statements that apply to you on the lists below. Add up the scores for each list and you will have a number for the plus score and one for the minus score. A high number on the 'plus' score indicates that you need to make changes to your lifestyle as your body is currently older than your years. A high number on the 'minus' score generally indicates you are on the right road and can take some years off your real age. If you do the simple calculation on page 57, you will find out your lifestyle age. It's as simple as that!

SECTION 1: STAYING YOUNGER

1 You generally feel in excellent health — 1 year ☐

2 You generally have a positive outlook on life — 1.5 years ☐

3 You rarely feel stressed — 1.5 years ☐

4 You take regular moderate walks of at least 30 minutes' duration five times per week (OR you do regular aerobic high intensity workouts of 20 minutes' duration two to three times per week) — 3 years ☐

5 You drink coffee sparingly or not at all — 0.5 years ☐

6 You drink 2 litres of water per day — 2 years ☐

7 You have never smoked — 3 years ☐

8 You never use salt, either in cooking or at the table — 1.5 years ☐

Subtotal: ▶

Subtotal carried forward: ____

____

9 You eat at least two portions of oily fish per week	−1 year	☐
10 You have regular health checks (blood pressure, cholesterol)	−0.5 years	☐
11 You usually eat low fat food	−1 year	☐
12 You generally have no more than one alcoholic drink per day	−3 years	☐
13 You do at least two strength training/ toning sessions per week	−1 year	☐
14 You eat breakfast every day	−1 year	☐
15 You always eat five portions of fruit and vegetables per day	−1.5 years	☐
16 You have no family history of heart disease, cancer or diabetes	−2 years	☐
17 You have on average seven hours' sleep per night	−1 year	☐
18 You have stayed an ideal weight for more than 10 years	−3 years	☐

____

Total 'minus' score: ____

SECTION 2: AGEING EARLY

1 You regularly feel low or depressed	+1 year	☐
2 You generally see the negative side of things	+1.5 years	☐
3 You frequently feel stressed	+2 years	☐
4 You take no regular exercise	+3 years	☐

5 You eat breakfast less than twice
per week   +1   year   ☐

6 You smoke more than one packet of
cigarettes per week   +5   years   ☐

7 You have been diagnosed with high
cholesterol or high blood pressure   +2   years   ☐

8 You rarely achieve five portions of
fruit and vegetables per day   +2   years   ☐

9 You are more than 2st overweight   +3   years   ☐
OR you are more than 4st overweight   +5   years   ☐

10 You have not visited a dentist in the
last 12 months   +1   year   ☐

11 You eat out or have takeaways more
than twice per week   +2   years   ☐

12 You drink more than 14 units of alcohol
per week (women) OR 21 units (men)   +5   years   ☐

13 You cook with fat in a chip pan/frying
pan more than once per week   +1.5 years   ☐

14 You regularly miss meals   +1.5 years   ☐

15 You regularly snack on high-fat foods
more than twice per day   +1.5 years   ☐

16 You regularly have disturbed sleep   +1   year   ☐

                                            ─────
                    Total 'plus' score:
                                            ─────

YOUR LIFESTYLE AGE REVEALED

Your age   = _____
Deduct your 'minus' score   = _____
Add your 'plus' score   = _____   = **Your lifestyle age**

Ten ways to make your lifestyle age younger

1 Reduce stress

In really stressful times your 'lifestyle' age can rocket upwards. Adopting stress-reducing strategies to help you through the difficult times can make a big difference. Exercise is a fantastic stress-buster, so try to incorporate more physical activity into your life. Seek help from others, including therapists, if stress is a major problem for you.

2 Stop smoking and avoid passive smoking

A smoker's skin wrinkles and dehydrates much more quickly than a non-smoker's due to the deprivation of oxygen caused through smoking. And that's what's showing on the outside. But what goes on in the inside is far more destructive and damaging, so it is not surprising that it adds to the ageing process. If you want to live to a good age, stopping smoking is a high priority.

3 Take regular exercise

We know so much now about the physical benefits of exercise. It will significantly help reduce symptoms of heart disease, aid diabetics, reduce stress, and keep us leaner and fitter. It really is a win/win situation. If you find formal exercise sessions difficult to fit in, then just be more active generally in your everyday life. Park further away from your destination, and use the stairs instead of the lift. Walk rather than drive to the shops, take up a sport or activity you used to enjoy when you were younger. Just get moving as it all adds up!

4 Be an ideal weight

The effects of being overweight can be hugely damaging to the body. Your whole system is in overdrive trying to cope with carrying the excess weight and causes you to age much more quickly. Overloading your joints, your heart and your whole body has serious health risks. Buying this book means that you have decided to do something, so let's start turning back the clock right now. It is never too late.

5 Eat low fat and low Gi

Eating a healthy, low-fat diet that is also low Gi really helps you lose weight. Eating less fat stops the whole system getting clogged up, which causes high blood pressure and high cholesterol levels, and eating low Gi stops you feeling hungry. Follow all the principles in this book and make what you have learned part of your lifestyle in the future, and you will have cracked it!

6 Reduce alcohol consumption

Not only is it high in calories, alcohol is also very toxic and damages major organs such as the liver. Alcohol also increases your appetite and dilutes your willpower, so be careful! However, a moderate consumption of one alcoholic drink per day is known to have health benefits – so it's not all bad news!

7 Eat more fruit and vegetables

Fruit and vegetables are packed with vitamins and minerals and eating plenty of these will ensure you have a great immune system to ward off illness and disease. Try to have as many different colours on your plate as you can. This will ensure you are taking in the whole range of vitamins and minerals. Aim to eat your five portions a day.

8 Drink more water

Dehydration is extremely ageing and nothing hydrates better than plain water. Avoid fizzy drinks, which can be full of chemicals.

9 Sleep well

We know that if we have had a good night's sleep we feel better. Make it a rule to go to bed at a reasonable time on most nights of the week and you will wake up refreshed and ready to cope more easily with what life throws at you! If you have a really late night, balance it out with an earlier one. Lack of sleep can be harmful to health.

10 Learn to think positive

A positive outlook on life, and smiling a lot, is good for us and helps us to live longer. Look back at this list and see how many things you can manage to do or improve. Start with one or two and gradually add some more. Be positive and make a commitment to those changes and you will soon reap tremendous benefits. If there is one message that comes through clearly from every successful slimmer that I meet, it is the increase in their confidence and self-esteem. And yes, you are worth it!

6 The secrets of slimming success

We don't suddenly wake up one day and realise we are over-weight. Those pounds of fat creep on over a matter of months, even years, until we reach the point when we say 'enough, is enough' and then we decide to do something about it. So here's what to do.

The principles of weight loss

Food comes in a vast variety of forms and some has much more fattening power than others. As I mentioned earlier, it's all to do with the 'energy value' of each individual food and this is measured in calories. Eat too many calories for your body's needs and you gain weight. Eat fewer calories than your body uses up each day and you will lose it. If you eat exactly the same number of calories that your body requires to function, your weight will remain constant. It's a delicate balance, but the good news is that by making informed choices about the type of foods you eat, you can lose weight without reducing the quantity of food you actually consume.

Cutting back on the calories

Fat (oil, butter, margarine, etc.) contains twice as many calories, gram for gram, as found in carbohydrate (rice, pasta, potatoes, bread and cereal) or protein (meat, fish, eggs, cheese and milk), so the obvious first step is to cut down on fat. Eating food with a maximum of five per cent fat (five grams of fat per 100 grams of food) will reduce your calorie intake dramatically without your having to eat less food.

Not being aware of the number of calories you are eating is a bit like not being aware of your bank balance. We all think we don't spend as much money as we actually do and we all think we eat less food and do more exercise than is often the case. The nicer the food tastes, the more likely we are to kid ourselves that we really are eating only a tiny portion, when in fact we're not!

Scientists have done trials on this very subject and found that, when trial subjects were given a free choice of foods to eat, they underestimated their portions by about a quarter! Further trials also showed that people overestimated their activity levels. So, in other words, many people don't understand why they are overweight because they think they eat less and physically do more than they actually do!

Calorie values give us an accurate means of measuring what we are actually consuming. My husband, Mike, and I normally eat a low-fat, healthy diet and manage to keep our weight reasonably stable, but we went on my Gi Jeans Kick-start Diet after returning from a rather overindulgent holiday with ample hips and very tight waistbands! I weighed out every portion carefully to ensure we didn't cheat. I also kept a written record of everything we ate and drank. I was shocked at the difference in portion sizes from what I normally dish up – and I thought those portions were modest! But the results were very rewarding. In two weeks I lost my excess 3lb and Mike lost the half stone he wanted to shed. The extra benefit from this exercise was the realisation that we actually felt perfectly satisfied with the smaller portions and vowed to eat a little less from then on!

Working out your calorie allowance

The number of calories we burn each day by just being alive is known as our basal metabolic rate (BMR) and this is dependent on a number of factors – our gender, age and weight. Men burn more calories than women do; the younger we are, the more calories we burn and, conversely, the older we are, the fewer we burn; the more we weigh, the more calories we use – rather like a car burns more fuel when it is carrying a heavier load. These are factors over which we have no control. We can, however, decide how much activity we do and this has a direct effect on the number of calories we burn each day. The more active we are, the more calories we spend.

The average woman will use around 1300–1500 calories a day simply in staying alive and for her body to keep functioning. Men will use around 1800–2000. As soon as you get out of bed and start going about your everyday tasks, you will inevitably burn more calories. If you are moving about you can't help but use extra calories, just as a car burns more fuel once it starts moving.

The key to successful, consistent weight loss, therefore, is to ensure that the body has enough calories to meet its basic metabolic needs, yet few enough to make it go 'overdrawn'. To make up the difference the body will automatically draw on its stores of fat to provide those extra calories to fuel any activity undertaken during each day. With sufficient calories each day (based on our BMR requirement), it is happy to allow its stored fat to supply the extra fuel required.

On my Ultimate Gi Jeans Diet, I recommend you follow the Kick-start Diet for the first two weeks. This has a daily allowance of 1200 calories. Then, after two weeks, you should move on to Part 2 of the diet, where your daily calorie allowance should be equal to your BMR. You can check this by referring to the BMR tables at the back of this book.

Checking the calorie value of foods

If you are following the diet in this book, then the calories in the menus have all been calculated for you. You can adjust your personal calorie allowance according to your BMR. If you stick to the meal suggestions as stated and weigh out your portions to ensure you don't overestimate your allowance, you will find it really easy.

When food shopping, check the label to find out the number of calories and how much fat a product contains. Quantities are always given per 100 grams of product, so just calculate the size of your portion and tot up the calories accordingly. You don't have to count up the fat grams if you only select foods with five per cent or less fat. It really isn't difficult once you realise the boundaries.

Effective exercise

Exercise burns extra calories and makes us fitter and healthier. It maximises our fat loss and also helps us keep the weight off. It also helps minimise any reduction in our BMR. Quite simply, exercise falls into two categories: aerobic and anaerobic. Aerobic means 'with oxygen' and describes exercise or activity where you breathe more deeply and cause your body to demand more oxygen into its bloodstream. This oxygen circulates around your body and calls on your fat stores to make fuel which then burns in your muscles. As well as being a fantastic fat burner, aerobic exercise encourages your skin to shrink as you lose weight because the blood circulation to your skin is so much better.

Anaerobic exercise, such as toning or strength exercises using weights or a resistance band, does not use oxygen to fuel the activity but instead specifically challenges the muscles to make them bigger and stronger and greatly improves our shape. The great news is that the stronger our muscles become, the more efficient they are in burning fat when we do aerobic exercise. So, try to combine both types of exercise – as we do at Rosemary Conley classes or on my DVDs – so that you get double the benefit.

And when people ask me 'Where does all the fat go?' I answer very simply that it just burns away into the atmosphere as heat, just like putting a log on the fire at home. So what are you waiting for?

Eat more for less

If you want to lose weight and eat healthily you need to eat less fat and fewer calories but that doesn't mean you have to reduce the quantity of food you eat. To speed up your weight-loss effortlessly here are some tips for cutting the calories and fat but not the quantity of food.

- Adding oil to your salads or food preparation means you are adding serious extra calories that you just don't need! All oil is 100 per cent fat. Try using a very-low-calorie dressing or use soy sauce or balsamic vinegar to dress your salads.

- If you use a non-stick frying pan or wok to cook your meals you don't need to add any fat. Providing the pan is hot when you add your raw chicken or meat, it will seal in the juices and keep them moist and tasty. You can dry-fry onions, peppers, mushrooms and save yourself literally hundreds of high-fat calories. Mushrooms and onions are like little sponges when cooked in fat, whether you cook with butter or oil. They will soak up the fat and transport it straight to your body, but it doesn't have to be that way if you dry-fry.

- Cooked basmati rice has 103 calories per 100 grams (that's around 35 grams uncooked weight rice) and we don't seem to get a lot of it for our portion when we are following a weight-reducing diet. Make it go further by adding fresh or canned beansprouts to your boiled rice. Beansprouts are low in fat and calories and they make a useful filler. They are also great in salads.

- Whenever you make a meat-based dish such as shepherd's or cottage pie, cut back on the quantity of meat and add some low-calorie grated vegetables, such as carrots or parsnips and chopped onions. It's also a great way to get your kids to eat more vegetables if they are not keen on eating them in the conventional way. No one will miss out on the portion size or the flavour, but you will cut out a lot of calories.

- Add some low-Gi beans and pulses to your casseroles and soups. Not only will they provide valuable low-fat protein, they will also make the meal more substantial and keep you feeling full for longer.

- If you usually serve cream or even crème fraîche with your dessert, switch to Normandy virtually fat free fromage frais instead. Double cream is 60 per cent fat and even single cream is 30 per cent fat. Crème fraîche varies but is usually around 38 per cent fat, or 17.5 per cent fat for the half-fat brands, which is still very high fat. Normandy fromage frais is much smoother than regular kinds and so tastes more luxurious, and you can easily find brands with less than five per cent fat. While natural yogurt is low fat I find it can be a bit thin as an accompaniment. Greek yogurt is thicker and creamier, so choose a brand with less than five per cent fat, or look for a premium organic yogurt, as these are generally thicker. They may be slightly more expensive but they are still cheaper than cream.
- The tomato is a great friend of the dieter. Low in fat and calories but high in health-giving antioxidants, tomatoes add versatility and taste to a vast variety of dishes. Whether bought fresh for salads or sandwiches, or canned, chopped or whole for cooking, liquefied as passata or concentrated as purée for sauces, tomatoes are good news! If you're in the supermarket wondering what sauce to pour on your pasta, go for a tomato-based one to save fat and calories.
- If you want to make a white sauce, rather than making a roux with butter and flour, use cornflour as a thickener instead. Whether it is a basic white sauce with onion, bay leaves and peppercorns, or something more exotic, just prepare a liquid base for the sauce with milk or stock and add flavourings in the usual way. Slake the cornflour with a little cold milk or water. Remove the unthickened sauce from the heat and slowly add the cornflour liquid to your sauce, stirring continually. Place back on a gentle heat and cook through for about

two minutes. You can still have a truly delicious sauce without adding butter!

- When preparing minced beef or lamb for a spaghetti bolognese or shepherd's pie, always dry-fry the meat first in a non-stick pan. When the meat changes colour, drain it through a colander to remove the liquid fat. All the fat that drains away is saving you heaps of calories and unwanted inches on your body.
- You can make delicious, low-fat sandwiches by spreading low-fat salad dressing or pickles straight on to your bread and cutting out the butter, margarine or low-fat spread all together. This will save you loads of unnecessary calories and your sandwiches will still taste delicious.

What about alcohol?

Most of us enjoy a drink, but how much is too much for our waistline and our health? Drinking too much alcohol is probably the most common reason why people find their rate of weight loss slow.

There's nothing like a drink to get you into the party mood at a special event or celebration and it has been medically proven that having a glass of wine every day is good for us. The problem comes because few people, having opened the bottle of cabernet sauvignon, stop at the one glass!

Maybe it's a long cool beer that takes your fancy, but these days the alcohol content of beers and lagers varies enormously, so you may be consuming more actual alcohol than you think. While a little alcohol is good, too much is very definitely bad for us. It can affect our general health as well as our life and work, family and friends, and, of course, it can significantly affect our weight-loss progress if we are on a weight-reducing diet.

One of the biggest drawbacks of drinking alcohol is that it can make you hungrier. Bad news for the dieter! You will find that you can keep eating for longer, that you can, after all, find a space for a pudding and then have a bit of a pick of the leftovers in the kitchen!

But there is no reason why we shouldn't enjoy the occasional drink. By understanding how the body deals with alcohol and by following a few simple rules we can still enjoy ourselves at a party or special celebration without piling on the pounds.

During normal digestion of food the body uses protein and carbohydrate as easy-to-burn fuel for energy, with fat only being burned for energy after the supplies of carbohydrate and protein we have consumed run out. However, alcohol is a toxin and as such the body works hard to eliminate it as soon as possible. Consequently the calories from alcohol suddenly go to the head of the queue and are burned off first, in preference to food.

The 'un-spent' food is then stored around the body and will be converted to fat, which causes weight gain. Only when you cut back the calories and increase your calorie expenditure with additional activity will those fat stores be reduced again so that your weight decreases once more.

During the two-week Kick-start Diet in this book you are asked to avoid alcohol for this short period. Once you embark on the main diet plan you are allowed 100 calories of alcohol each day and you can save up your allowance for a special event.

So, if you enjoy a tipple here's how to help limit any damage.

Keep to your limits

Women should restrict their alcohol intake to a maximum of 14 units a week, and men 21 units. One unit equates to one small glass of wine, a single measure of spirits or 300ml (½ pint) of regular lager or beer.

Give your body a break

Unless you can restrict your alcohol consumption to one or two units a day you need to have 'rest days' from your drinking. It is really bad for your general health if you have a lot to drink very regularly. Your work performance will be affected, your weight-loss progress will probably be zero and you won't feel like exercising.

Take more water with it

As the size of wine glasses and the strength of alcohol in some wines and beers increases it becomes even more difficult to judge exactly how much we are drinking. One of the best tips on an evening out is to alternate each glass of wine with a glass of water. It will keep you hydrated, which will help prevent the alcohol going straight to your head, and it will definitely help you to drink less wine.

Get on the dance floor

If you are at a disco or party, get up and dance whenever you can. While you are on the dance floor you are not only not drinking but you are very effectively burning lots of extra calories. Dancing is a great fat-burner as well as fun.

Don't go for a curry when you leave your party!

Alcohol not only makes you feel hungry, it makes you want to eat high-fat food. Going for a curry on top of a very social night will not only lay heavily in your stomach, it will make you feel dreadful through the night and as though you've swallowed an elephant the next morning. It's just not worth it.

Alcohol can certainly have a place within a calorie-controlled, healthy diet. Keep your intake to a moderate level and it acts as a valuable relaxant and makes a social event more enjoyable. As with all things, moderation is the key, particularly when you are trying to lose weight.

CALORIES IN ALCOHOL

Beer and cider (per 300ml/½ pint)

Beer or bitter	85
Sweet cider	120
Dry cider	100
Lager	85
Low-alcohol lager	35
Strong lager	170

Liqueurs (per 25ml pub measure)

Advocat	65
Cointreau	78
Grand Marnier	78
Irish cream	81
Tia Maria	65

Spirits (per 25ml pub measure)

Brandy	50
Gin	50
Rum	50
Vodka	50
Whisky	50

continued

Sherry (per 50ml pub measure)

Dry and medium sherry	60
Sweet sherry	80

Wine (per 150ml)

Red	100
Dry white	100
Sparkling white	120
Sweet white	140

Ten foolproof ways to speed up your weight loss

Once you decide to lose weight you want to see results fast! Here are my top ten tips to help speed up your progress.

1 Write it down

Actually putting pen to paper to record what you eat has a dramatic effect on your discipline when following a calorie-controlled eating plan. It makes you think before you eat that extra sweet or chocolate or drink that extra glass of wine. But the key is to record everything you eat and drink as you consume it, and not at the end of the day when you will have, perhaps not intentionally, forgotten half of what you had!

2 Weigh it out

Portions can be deceptive so use your weighing scales to check exactly how much cereal/rice/pasta you are actually serving to yourself. If you stick to the eating plan strictly, your excess weight will fall away. Cheat – and it won't!

3 Get moving!

When you sit down you use half the number of calories compared with when you are standing, and a quarter the number compared to when you are walking, so be aware that being more active generally will greatly speed up your weight-loss progress. Do get yourself a pedometer and try to achieve 10,000 steps a day. It's not easy to do that many at first, but with a few changes in your day-to-day lifestyle it is very achievable. I try to do it and on six days out of seven I achieve it. The great thing about wearing a pedometer is the fact that it makes you much more aware of trying to be more active.

4 Exercise, exercise, exercise!

If you want to lose weight fast, get exercising. Doing any form of exercise that makes you breathe more deeply BURNS FAT! Once you have warmed up for aerobic exercise, for say five minutes, you will be entering into 'fat burning mode'. Keep exercising for another 20 minutes at a rate that makes you a bit breathless and warm, and you are into serious fat burning. Then cool down with less energetic moves and some stretches and you will feel fantastic. It will give you a real boost to how you feel as well as dramatically help to speed up your weight loss.

5 Turn yourself into a fat burner

Exercising aerobically on a regular basis will help you create more mitochondria (little engines) in your muscles. If you have fit and strong muscles, you automatically turn your body into a fat-burning machine, which means that even when you are not exercising you will be *burning* rather than *storing* fat as you go about your everyday work. This is such good news for weight maintenance once you reach your goal.

6 Don't cheat!

When you eat or drink something extra to your calorie allowance, you are only cheating yourself. If you want to lose weight fast and continuously, stick to your calorie allowance. Realise that if you ate just one chocolate digestive biscuit every day for a year on top of what you normally eat you would gain 12lb in 12 months!

7 Cook without fat

With non-stick pans it is really simple to cook everything you need without adding fat or oil to the pan or to recipes. I never cook with oil or any form of fat and personally hate the taste of it when dining out. It doesn't take long to change your taste buds and it is the quickest and surest way to cut down on hundreds of calories without even affecting the portion size. Remember, fat that you eat becomes fat on your body, so cut it right down and you can avoid 'replacing' the fat you are burning off during aerobic exercise and just get leaner!

8 Eat the low-Gi way

Low-Gi foods are filling and satisfying. They are good for your health and your appetite as they help you feel fuller for longer thus avoiding the temptation to snack on high-fat, high calorie, foods between meals – the downfall of most dieters. Learning the Gi values of foods can be complicated and often contradictory as different brands of a similar food often have different values. Following the guidelines contained in this book makes it really simple. You don't have to be a slave to Gi. Just eating more low-Gi foods than you used to within your daily diet will give you a real health boost and will satisfy your hunger.

9 Prepare your own food

We all know that a busy lifestyle and lack of time can cause us to dive into the ready-meal section at the supermarket, but cooking your own food needn't be difficult or too time-consuming. Try the recipes in this book. You'll find them really easy to prepare. Also, give some ready-made sauces a try as, combined with some dry-fried meat or poultry and some cooked pasta, a meal can be prepared in minutes to satisfy the fussiest of families. By cooking it yourself, you can make the meal more nutritious and usually much more satisfying. You could involve the children in the preparation of the dish and help them to learn about healthy cooking.

10 Attention alcohol!

While drinking alcohol in moderation can be good for us, if drunk in excess it is definitely bad for us! Alcohol not only weakens our willpower, it also increases our appetite, so drink with caution if you want to see your weight disappear quickly! Alcohol is also dehydrating, which is also unhelpful. I know everyone tells us to drink more water but it IS good for our health.

7 The miracle of a shrinking body

If we have a large amount of weight to lose, when we embark on a weight-reducing diet, a big worry is that we will be left with lots of excess skin. This needn't be the case if we go about it the right way.

Where we store most of our fat depends on our body type. Broadly speaking we tend to be one of three shapes: apple, pear or heart. An 'apple' will store most of her fat on her stomach, a 'pear' on her hips and thighs, and a 'heart' on her chest. A woman who weighs 16st and who would describe herself as an 'apple' shape will undoubtedly be carrying a great deal of fat on her stomach. But this does NOT mean she would be left with lots of excess skin if she lost weight, providing she took the right approach to her weight-loss programme.

If she were to follow a healthy low-fat diet that offered a calorie allowance appropriate to her gender, age and weight and initially combined with gentle aerobic exercise such as walking and some muscle-strengthening exercises, there is no reason why the skin shouldn't shrink back amazingly well. It would probably be unrealistic to imagine that it would shrink back completely to achieve a washboard stomach, but there's a huge amount that can be done to maximise its reduction. Here's how:

1 Eat enough

The worst thing you can do is to go on a crash diet of, say, 800 calories as this will cause a too rapid weight loss and not help the skin at all. Instead, if you follow the Ultimate Gi Jeans Diet plan in this book, its two-week Kick-start plan of 1200 calories will get you off to a great start and you can then move on to a more generous calorie allowance. For a lady in her mid-40s who weighs, say, 16st, I recommend a daily allowance of around 1673 calories. This is equal to her basal metabolic rate (BMR) – the number of calories she needs each day for her body to function. Then every bit of activity she does will burn fat from her body. As her weight decreases, she should reduce her daily allowance a little, so when she gets down to, say, 11st, she should be eating around 1400 calories.

2 Check with your doctor

Carrying a great deal of excess weight can restrict mobility because the joints struggle to cope with the load, and the heart has to work extremely hard each time we start to move about energetically. So check with your doctor to see if you can start some gentle exercise without putting your health at risk.

3 Get walking!

You need to do some aerobic exercise, such as walking, which will burn fat as fuel – just what you want. What's more, the increased oxygen that your body forces into your bloodstream will also reach your skin, which will help it to shrink. All of this is key to helping your stomach reduce in size and shrink back. Start gently by walking 100–200 metres a couple of times a day and gradually increase the distance. When you are coping more easily, try one of my fitness videos or DVDs – don't attempt the whole workout yet, but just do the warm-up. As you become fitter, progress to the next track. Before you finish, always fast-forward to the cool-down stretches and do these.

4 Get toning!

To help increase the fat-burning effect, you also need to strengthen your muscles, particularly the abdominal muscles. The fat that we burn during exercise is only burned in the muscles and the bigger the muscles, the more effective the fat burning. If you are significantly overweight, lying down on the floor can be uncomfortable and doing abdominal exercises may be difficult. Try using a rolled-up towel under your head for support.

5 Get creaming

I am not for a moment suggesting that applying a cream to your skin is going to work miracles, because it won't, but there are two real benefits from applying some kind of body lotion every day after your bath or shower. When our skin is significantly stretched, say during pregnancy or through being seriously over-weight, we are challenging its elasticity. By applying a moisturising body lotion, or even baby oil, we help to keep the skin soft and more pliable. In addition to the replacement of important moisture, the very act of applying the lotion also massages the skin and helps improve circulation. This is another aid to encourage the skin to shrink back when we lose weight.

Follow these five simple steps and you should lose 2–3lb each week. As you become slimmer and fitter, increase your activity. Investing just 20–30 minutes on five days a week could save your life, let alone the cost of cosmetic surgery!

8 Go for goal

We find ourselves wanting to lose weight at different times of our lives for a variety of reasons and summoning up the motivation to achieve our goals isn't easy.

An important forthcoming event such as a wedding where we will be photographed for lots to view provides the perfect reason to focus our minds and make the effort. Or it might be a special invitation to an important function such as a school reunion, where how we look really matters and we want to look our absolute best.

Another great motivator is a summer holiday. There's nothing quite like imagining ourselves on the beach in a bikini, or even shorts, to make us go hot and cold with dread at what we might look like if we don't take action right now! And what happens on holiday? We take photos!

But what do we do if there is no holiday, school reunion or family wedding on the horizon? How do we give ourselves that kick up the backside?

Know yourself

Maybe we should spend some time getting to know ourselves better and what motivates us as individuals. Think carefully about the reasons WHY you WANT to lose weight and write them all down in a notebook or diary to act as a reminder. Seeing your reasons on paper makes it more real and will hopefully help motivate you into action.

Recently I have been reading Professor Raj Persaud's most excellent book *The Motivated Mind* (Bantam Press), which I found totally fascinating. If you are interested in learning about how we tick – and there's plenty on the subject of trying to lose weight or becoming fitter – you will realise that how successful we are in losing weight depends to a great degree on our personality type.

Various studies have been carried out with the apparent conclusion that if you are a 'live your life for today' kind of person, which apparently most overweight people are, you are likely to want to eat that cream cake now because you aren't too worried about tomorrow, anyway. You may not be able to imagine yourself slim with all the pleasure that it hopefully will bring you, but you are very certain of the pleasure you will get in eating that cake!

A forward thinking type of person is more likely to be concerned about their future health and motivated to take action before it's too late. Alternatively, you might be someone who is always looking back and maybe remembering a time when you used to be a size 10 and want to go back there but don't quite understand why it's so tough now. Our lifestyles change as we get older and with those changes we probably do less and eat more as no doubt we have different eating habits, probably dining out more now than then.

I am fascinated by people and, as a creator of diet plans and a teacher of exercise, it is challenging to come up with a variety of solutions to appeal to the many and varied personality types that are obviously around. Every one of us, of course, is unique, with different strengths and weaknesses and I believe the key is learning more about ourselves and understanding what works best for us as individuals.

There is no doubt that some people find it easier than others to stick to a diet and this depends upon our motivation and our willpower. Some of us are just weak if offered a favourite treat while others are rigid in their determination with the inevitable greater reward for their unfaltering resolve. Some people enjoy attending classes and interacting with folks just like them, but others feel they couldn't cope with a class situation. It is for that very reason that I launched my online slimming club. It suits people who want to be very private in their weight-loss campaign or who maybe wake up in the middle of the night and need support from other nocturnal members with whom they can communicate and empathise if they wish through the online coffee shop.

Still another type is the lone-dieter who just wants to do it on their own and the Rosemary Conley at-home Postal Pack provides all the tools – diet, DVDs, charts, etc. – for people to go it alone.

But for any of these to work I believe the key is to look inside our personality and be honest about our sensitivities. We all need encouragement and recognition of our success. It's human nature and we need to find someone who will be an encourager and a comforter and, also ideally, an 'exercise buddy'. If that person can be your partner, that's ideal. You are together more than you are likely to be with anyone else and to have your partner noticing and encouraging your progress is perfect. If you don't have a supportive partner, find a close friend or relative to help instead.

Then, once you have decided who is going to fulfil that role, you need to decide how closely you are going to allow them in to your dieting campaign. Will you let them weigh and even perhaps measure you? If you're thinking 'You've got to be joking!' then ask yourself if you will even tell them what you weigh. You may feel too embarrassed to share such private information and if that is the case, that's fine, but do plan how you are going to communicate your progress. Some prospective dieters can't face knowing this information themselves, let alone discuss it with a partner, but they may be happy for a class instructor to know because that's their job. Think about it so that you are aware of your personal boundaries before you start enlisting support.

Plan ahead

Once you've made your decision to start losing weight and becoming fitter, discuss your plan with your 'weight mate'. Then set out some goals about timescales. Let's imagine it is early February and you want to lose a stone (14lb) by the end of March. This is very achievable if you stick strictly to the diet in this book.

To ensure you achieve this goal you need to plan your exercise sessions – ideally five sessions a week of aerobic activity and two or three toning sessions (see the Ultimate Gi Jeans Diet workout in chapter 15). Make an exercise plan to ensure you find the time to actually do it. We can be full of great intentions sitting on the sofa late on a Sunday evening planning the week ahead, but when we come home from work two days later, tired and stressed, exercise just doesn't feel attractive but the glass or two of wine does! But if you have made an 'appointment' with your exercise buddy that at six o'clock you are going for a walk or are going to work out to a fitness video or are going to a class that evening, it is much harder to back out. We don't want to appear as though we are faltering and we don't want to let our friend down either. Fortunately, there is nothing like exercise for neutralising stress and turning pent-up, negative feelings into positive ones. It is just the best thing to do if you've had a hard day at work.

Next, set a day each week for your weigh-in and measuring session. Again, if your partner or best friend can be part of this, all the better. It is a golden opportunity to receive lots of encouragement as your weight and inches fall away. Obviously if you can get to a class, that determines your weigh-in timetable and measuring yourself at the class can be extremely motivational as you can share your good news with lots of people who feel just like you and want to share in your success.

The next bit of planning involves your food shopping. Make a plan of meals you intend to cook throughout the week and make a list of which foods you need to buy to achieve this. If you are planning to dine out, think carefully about what you are going to eat and what type of restaurant will best suit your needs while trying to lose weight. Try to limit your meals out if possible to reduce the risk of overindulgence. It is much harder to be disciplined when there are so many delicious options on offer and even the most dedicated dieter will struggle after drinking a couple of glasses of wine!

Chart your progress

Remember to chart your progress, recording your measurements as well as your weight (see the charts at the back of this book), and then get an old carrier bag and place in it some out-of-date tins or packets equal to the weight you lose each week. Allow them to accumulate each week so you will never forget how much weight you are losing. This is hugely motivating. Also, find an old tape measure, or draw one on a piece of paper, and colour in how many inches you lose each week so that you can see those inches or centimetres extending too. There is nothing as motivating as seeing the physical evidence equal to your progress. Please make the effort and do this as it really does work.

Celebrate your success!

Finally, promise yourself a reward each time you lose a stone. Plan for it together with your weight mate and celebrate together if you can. We all need to feel needed and it's great when the valuable support you have been given is acknowledged. It becomes a team effort where everybody wins. You feel healthier and happier and your 'supporter' feels appreciated. Perfect!

9 How to use the Ultimate Gi Jeans Diet programme

The Ultimate Gi Jeans Diet is divided into two parts. Part 1 is the Gi Jeans Kick-start Diet, which is strict but lasts for only two weeks. It is designed to give an initial boost to your weight-loss progress, which will then motivate you to carry on.

In week three, you move on to Part 2 of the Ultimate Gi Jeans Diet, which has a much more generous calorie allowance. It allows you 100 calories of alcohol, two low-fat, low-Gi Power Snacks each day to eat between meals plus a daily treat worth 100 calories, which can be anything you like as it is outside the low-fat and low-Gi guidelines. And the good news is that you can save up your alcohol allowance *and* your treats over several days to accommodate a social occasion or special event. This versatility enables the diet to fit in with your lifestyle and gives you ultimate freedom while you reduce your weight and discover the new, slimmer, healthier you that's dying to get out!

No need to count calories, fat or Gi values

All the meal suggestions are calorie-counted, Gi aware and low in fat. Each meal category states the calorie content and you can choose which meals you like, repeat your favourites and avoid those that don't take your fancy.

This diet will work best if you are happy with what you are eating. If you really cannot face a high-fibre, natural grain cereal every morning and feel you could only survive on the diet by eating your favourite cereal for breakfast, for instance a high-Gi one such as Rice Krispies or cornflakes, then have it. The idea is to incorporate more low-Gi foods into your daily diet than you used to so that your overall diet is much healthier. Even if you substitute your own meal ideas in place of the ones listed, so long as you stick to the calorie allowance and observe the five per cent fat rule, the diet will still work.

Eating low-Gi foods alone will not make you lose weight faster, but it will keep you feeling fuller for longer so you are less likely to snack. The low-fat, low-Gi Power Snacks that are allowed mid-morning and mid-afternoon each day are designed to stave off hunger pangs so that your tendency to snack throughout the day on high-fat foods such as chocolates, crisps and biscuits can be controlled, which will enable you to stay on track.

Lose weight faster

Remember, if you want to see fast results and watch your skin shrink back and your muscle tone reappear, you will need to take some form of physical activity or exercise at least five times a week. This needn't be arduous or excessive – it is just about being on the go more and sitting down watching TV less. It is important for you to understand which exercise does what, and that is covered in chapter 14. Please take the time to read it if you are serious about losing weight faster and achieving a fit and healthy body.

Lifestyle changes

The only way you are going to manage to lose your excess weight and keep it off in the long term is by re-educating your eating habits and making some lifestyle changes that will really help you stay fit and slim without a huge amount of effort. This is not a 'boot camp' regimen. It is an easy, effective and enjoyable journey towards a new you!

As one of the trial dieters wrote: 'I can't believe how healthy and fit I feel. I've gone down three dress sizes – I recently bought size 10 trousers. I haven't worn size 10 for 20 years!'

Get started

So, you are ready to start the Ultimate Gi Jeans Kick-start Diet. Read through it carefully to understand how it works and what foods you need to purchase (and which ones you don't!).

The results from my trial dieters (see chapter 2) should provide all the encouragement you need to give it your best shot. Weight losses of up to 14lb in the first two weeks were not uncommon, although 7lb was the average in the initial trial. In the more extensive, later trial, the average weight loss over eight weeks was one and a half stone! Can you imagine what a difference that could make to how your clothes fit? Enjoy the results.

Reading nutrition labels

The nutrition label on each food product we buy provides a breakdown of its nutritional content as well as the number of calories and amount of fat. To simplify matters, as far as weight control is concerned, the two key things to look at are the 'energy' and the 'fat' values.

The figure relating to 'energy' tells you the number of calories (kcal) in 100 grams of the product (you can ignore the kj figure). You then need to calculate how much of the product you will actually be eating to work out the number of *calories per portion*.

NUTRITIONAL INFORMATION

	Per 100g
ENERGY	172kj/40 kcal
PROTEIN	1.8g
CARBOHYDRATE	8.0g
(of which sugars)	(2.0g)
FAT	0.2g
(of which saturates)	(Trace)
FIBRE	1.5g
SODIUM	0.3g

The fat content may be broken down into polyunsaturated and saturated but, for anyone on a weight-reducing diet, it is the total fat content per 100 grams that is the most significant. Remember, when following my Ultimate Gi Jeans Diet you should only select foods where the label shows the fat content as five grams or less per 100 grams weight of product. The actual amount of fat per portion is of lesser importance. If you follow the simple five per cent fat rule and restrict your calorie intake to around 1400–1500 calories a day for women and 1700–2000 calories a day for men, depending on your age and current weight, the fat content of your food will look after itself. The only exceptions to this rule are oily fish, such as salmon, herring and mackerel, which may yield as much as 10 per cent fat. Also, some lean cuts of meat and some brands of wholegrain bread may be just over the five per cent yardstick. These are allowed on this diet because of the important nutrients they contain.

Remember that, although the five per cent rule is the ideal while you are trying to lose weight, I accept that you might crave a high-fat treat or dine out and be unable to control what foods you eat. That's why, in Part 2 of the Ultimate Gi Jeans Diet, I have included a daily treat, which can be outside the low-fat, low-Gi guidelines and which can be saved up if you wish. The occasional high-fat treat is not a disaster. The key is to enjoy it and not to resort to a binge. Just try to balance the calories.

If you wonder why I recommend the five per cent fat rule rather than counting the actual fat grams in a portion, it is because I want to educate people to adopt low-fat eating as a lifestyle habit. If you were to start counting fat grams per portion you could include lots of relatively unhealthy foods that would keep your taste buds requiring more. If, on the other hand you learn which foods are low fat and steer your eating in that direction you will be much more likely to maintain your new weight in the long term.

10 The Ultimate Gi Jeans Kick-start Diet

Follow this Kick-start Diet for two weeks only to give you a head start in your weight-loss campaign. Remember to cook and serve all foods without adding fat. Grill or dry-fry foods instead of frying (or use a little spray oil) and cook vegetables, rice and pasta in water with a vegetable stock cube for added flavour.

What to do

Each day, select one breakfast, lunch and dinner menu. You can repeat any of the menu options as you wish to suit your taste and lifestyle. You should also consume 450ml (¾ pint) skimmed or semi-skimmed milk. If you prefer, you may substitute a low-fat, low-calorie yogurt (max. 75 calories) for 150ml (¼ pint) milk. Tea and coffee can be drunk freely, using milk from your allowance

In addition to the breakfast, lunch and dinner menus you are allowed two extra pieces of fruit as Power Snacks. You may substitute 120ml (4fl oz) fruit juice for one of your fruit options.

These Power Snacks should be eaten mid-morning and mid-afternoon. You are also allowed $1 \times 175g$ (6oz) extra portion of salad each day, which can be eaten with lunch or dinner or as a separate snack

For good health, aim to incorporate five portions of vegetables and/or fruit each day in your daily allowance. These will also help fill you up and help you to lose weight faster.

During this two-week Kick-start Diet do not drink any alcohol but do drink at least five large glasses of water each day. Don't worry – after the two weeks are completed you can drink alcohol again!

I always recommend that anyone who follows a weight-reducing diet take a multi-vitamin supplement but it is particularly important during this stricter two-week diet.

So to recap, each day you can have:

Breakfast	200 kcal
Mid-morning Power Snack	50 kcal
Lunch	250 kcal
Mid-afternoon Power Snack	50 kcal
Dinner	400 kcal
Extra portion of salad	50 kcal
450ml (¾ pint) skimmed or semi-skimmed milk	200 kcal
Unlimited tea and coffee	
At least 5 large glasses of water	
	Total 1200 kcal

Diet notes

Low fat

The term 'low fat' refers to any product with five per cent or less fat.

Bread

Bread should be stoneground, multigrain or wholegrain. For ease of reference within the diet plan, one slice should contain no more than 125 calories.

Breakfast cereals

Try to choose whole-oat or high-fibre varieties, e.g. All-Bran, Fruit 'n Fibre, Bran Buds, Grapenuts, muesli, Shredded Wheat. Special K is also low Gi, and Weetabix is a good low-fat, low-sugar option.

Fruit

'1 piece fruit' means one apple, one pear, etc., or 115g (4oz) fruit such as grapes, strawberries, etc. For the purposes of this diet, one banana counts as two pieces. Choose slightly under-ripe bananas rather than over-ripe ones for a lower Gi rating.

Salad

'Salad' includes all salad leaves, cress, tomatoes and raw vegetables such as cucumber, peppers, carrots, onion, mushrooms, celery and courgettes, and may be served with 2 tsps fat-free, low-calorie dressing.

Drinks

Drink plenty of water, at least five large glasses a day. Don't drink any alcohol for the two weeks of the Ultimate Gi Jeans Kick-start Diet. Tea and coffee may be drunk freely, using milk from your allowance. Low-calorie and 'diet' drinks are also permissable.

Milk

Milk can be skimmed or semi-skimmed, cow's, goat's or soya milk. If you find 450ml (¾ pint) is too much, you can always substitute a low-fat yogurt in place of 150ml (¼ pint) milk. This can be eaten as a dessert or as a between-meal snack if you wish.

You will find further menu ideas and meal suggestions in my original *Gi Jeans Diet*.

Ⓥ means suitable for vegetarians or vegetarian option is available.

Breakfasts

Approx. 200 kcal each. Select one per day.

CEREAL BREAKFASTS

- Ⓥ 2 Weetabix served with milk from allowance and 2 tsps sugar; 1 kiwi fruit
- Ⓥ 40g (1½oz) any whole-oat or high-fibre cereal served with 1 tsp sugar and milk from allowance; 1 piece fruit
- Ⓥ 20g (¾oz) any whole-oat or high-fibre cereal served with milk from allowance and low-calorie sweetener; 1 × 100g pot low-fat fruit yogurt (max. 75 kcal) and 1 piece fruit
- Ⓥ 40g (1½oz) Sultana Bran Flakes served with milk from allowance, 1 sliced peach or nectarine and 1 tbsp 0% fat Greek-style yogurt (e.g. Total 0%)
- Ⓥ 20g (¾oz) Special K cereal served with milk from allowance; ½ slice toasted wholegrain bread spread with Marmite and topped with 10 grilled cherry tomatoes; 1 piece fruit
- Ⓥ 40g (1½oz) unsweetened muesli topped with 1 chopped apple or pear and served with milk from allowance
- Ⓥ 40g (1½oz) unsweetened muesli soaked overnight in 100ml (3½fl oz) unsweetened apple juice and topped with 1 tsp very low fat natural yogurt
- Ⓥ 40g (1½oz) porridge oats cooked in water and served with milk from allowance and 1 tsp runny honey or sugar

FRUIT BREAKFASTS

- Ⓥ 1 large banana, sliced, served with 1 pot low-fat yogurt (max. 100 kcal)
- Ⓥ Gi fruit salad comprising 1 satsuma, broken into segments, 1 pear, finely chopped with skin intact, 25g (1oz) seedless grapes and 15g (½oz) oats mixed with 2 tbsps 0% fat Greek-style yogurt (e.g. Total 0%)
- Ⓥ 4 pieces fruit (excluding bananas)
- Ⓥ 2 pieces fruit plus 1 medium banana or 1 pot low-fat yogurt (max. 75 kcal)
- Ⓥ 225g (8oz) fresh fruit topped with 2 tbsps 0% fat Greek-style yogurt (e.g. Total 0%)
- Ⓥ ½ small melon, any type, filled with 115g (4oz) raspberries and topped with 1 pot low-fat yogurt (max. 100 kcal)
- Ⓥ Summer Berry Smoothie (see recipe, page 264); 1 × 35g Rosemary Conley Low Gi Nutrition Bar

QUICK AND EASY BREAKFASTS

- Ⓥ 1 Muller Fruit Corner yogurt plus 10 chopped strawberries
- Ⓥ 1 × 35g Rosemary Conley Low Gi Nutrition Bar, plus 1 low-fat yogurt (max. 85 kcal)
- Ⓥ 1 slice toasted wholegrain bread spread with 2 tsps honey or marmalade; 1 piece fruit
- Ⓥ Cheese on toast: 1 slice toasted wholegrain bread spread with 1 level tsp chutney, then topped with 25g (1oz) low-fat Cheddar cheese and grilled until golden and bubbling; 1 piece fruit

continued

- Ⓥ Pizza toastie: 1 slice toasted wholegrain bread covered with sliced ripe tomatoes, then topped with 25g (1oz) sliced half-fat mozzarella cheese and grilled until melted; 115g (4oz) fresh raspberries or strawberries served with 1 low-fat yogurt (max. 75 kcal)

COOKED BREAKFASTS

- Ⓥ 1 fresh grapefruit sprinkled with low-calorie sweetener if desired; 1 medium-sized boiled egg served with ½ slice toasted wholegrain bread spread with Marmite
- 1 slice wholegrain bread spread with savoury sauce, e.g. tomato ketchup, fruity sauce, etc., and topped with 2 grilled turkey rashers; 1 piece fruit
- 50g (2oz) smoked salmon and 1 medium-sized scrambled egg
- Ⓥ 1½ slices toasted wholegrain bread topped with 1 × 200g can tomatoes boiled until thick and reduced
- Ⓥ 1 medium slice toasted wholegrain bread topped with 1 × 150g can baked beans
- Ⓥ 1 slice toasted wholegrain bread topped with 3 tbsps baked beans and 2 sliced tomatoes
- 1 medium-sized egg, poached or dry-fried, served with 1 grilled low-fat sausage, 4 grilled tomatoes and 115g (4oz) grilled mushrooms
- Ⓥ ½ pink grapefruit; 1 medium-sized poached egg served on 1 slice toasted wholegrain bread

Lunches

Approx. 250 kcal each. Select one per day.

SANDWICH AND SNACK LUNCHES

- 1 medium slice wholegrain bread spread with sauce of your choice, and topped with 50g (2oz) wafer thin turkey or chicken and 1 tsp cranberry sauce, plus unlimited salad
- 1 slice wholegrain bread spread with 25g (1oz) extra light cream cheese and topped with 50g (2oz) smoked salmon plus cherry tomatoes and salad leaves
- Ⓥ 2 slices wholegrain bread spread with low-calorie, reduced-fat salad dressing and filled with unlimited salad vegetables plus 25g (1oz) wafer thin ham/chicken/beef or 50g (2oz) low-fat cottage cheese
- Ⓥ 1 × 50g wholegrain baguette rubbed with a cut garlic clove, toasted, and topped with 50g (2oz) wafer thin pastrami or low-fat cottage cheese and unlimited salad tossed in oil-free vinaigrette dressing
- 1 wholemeal tortilla wrap spread with sweet chilli sauce and filled with chopped peppers, red onion, celery, cherry tomatoes, cucumber, salad leaves and 25g (1oz) shredded wafer thin ham
- 1 × 50g (2oz) pitta bread filled with shredded salad leaves, cherry tomatoes, 25g (1oz) flaked salmon and 1 tbsp 0% fat Greek-style yogurt (e.g. Total 0%) mixed with 1 tsp tomato ketchup and black pepper; 1 piece fruit

continued

- Ⓥ Mixed Pepper Bruschetta (see recipe, page 222) served with a large mixed salad; 1 kiwi fruit
- 1 × 50g (2oz) pitta bread filled with 50g (2oz) crab meat, chopped spring onions, shredded lettuce, chopped fresh coriander and a squeeze of lemon juice
- Ⓥ 1 × 50g (2oz) pitta bread filled with shredded lettuce, sliced peppers, spring onions, tomatoes and either 50g (2oz) canned salmon in brine or 50g (2oz) low-fat cottage cheese mixed with 1 tbsp sweetcorn
- Ⓥ 1 mini pitta bread served with Lemon and Mustard Seed Humous (see recipe, page 244)
- 3 Ryvita Dark Rye crispbreads spread with Marmite and topped with 75g (3oz) low-fat cottage cheese; 1 apple, pear or orange
- Ⓥ Any prepacked low-fat sandwich (max. 250 kcal)

SALAD LUNCHES
- 50g (2oz) wafer thin ham, chicken or beef or 75g (3oz) low-fat cottage cheese served with a large salad; Blueberry Syllabub (see recipe, page 262)
- Ⓥ Chickpea salad: mix 115g (4oz) drained, canned chickpeas with chopped peppers, cherry tomatoes and baby spinach leaves, and toss in oil-free dressing. Add a squeeze of lemon juice, and garnish with chopped fresh basil and mint leaves; 1 pot low-fat yogurt (max. 75 kcal)

continued

- 50g (2oz) salmon, mackerel or trout served with 1 tsp horseradish sauce and a large salad tossed in oil-free dressing; 1 medium banana
- 50g (2oz) skinned and boned, cooked chicken breast, chopped and mixed with 1 tbsp low-fat plain yogurt, 1 tbsp mango chutney, then piled on to 2 Ryvita Dark Rye crispbreads and served with cherry tomatoes, chunks of cucumber, celery sticks and mixed salad leaves
- 115g (4oz) [cooked weight] pasta shapes mixed with 50g (2oz) drained canned tuna in brine, chopped spring onions, cucumber, tomato and 1 tbsp sweetcorn kernels plus 2 tbsps low-calorie salad dressing
- Ⓥ 350g (12oz) chopped salad vegetables (e.g. peppers, onions, tomatoes, cucumber, celery, carrots, baby sweetcorn) sprinkled with soy sauce or balsamic vinegar to taste, plus 1 chicken drumstick (all skin removed) or 1 × 200g can baked beans (served cold); 1 piece fruit
- Ⓥ Salad leaves, sliced peppers and cherry tomatoes topped with 115g (4oz) low-fat cottage cheese mixed with 75g (3oz) low-fat coleslaw; 1 piece fruit
- Ⓥ Fruity lentil salad: 150g (5oz) cooked brown lentils mixed with 2 chopped spring onions, 1 chopped sun-dried tomato, 2 chopped fresh apricots and herbs, tossed in oil-free dressing and topped with 1 tbsp virtually fat free fromage frais
- Ⓥ Any prepacked low-fat salad (max. 250 kcal)

COOKED LUNCHES

- ⓥ 1 slice toasted wholegrain bread topped with 1 poached or dry-fried egg and served with 3 grilled tomatoes; 1 piece fresh fruit
- ⓥ Super-quick stir-fry: preheat a non-stick pan or wok till hot. Add 150g (5oz) skinned and boned chicken breast or 225g (8oz) Quorn chunks and plenty of freshly ground black pepper and dry-fry until thoroughly cooked. Add 350g (12oz) chopped vegetables (ideally include some beansprouts) and dry-fry until hot. Sprinkle with 2 tbsps soy sauce and toss to lightly coat the vegetables. Serve immediately
- ⓥ Stir-fry Quorn (see recipe, page 241) served with 40g (1½oz) [uncooked weight] boiled basmati rice
- 2 low-fat sausages, grilled, served on 1 slice toasted wholegrain bread with 1 × 200g can tomatoes boiled until thick and reduced; 1 piece fruit
- ⓥ 1 × 175g (6oz) sweet potato baked in its skin and topped with 100g (3½oz) low-fat plain cottage cheese mixed with 1 tsp chilli sauce, 15g (½oz) finely chopped red onion, and ¼ each chopped red, green and yellow peppers
- ⓥ 1 can low-fat soup (max. 150 kcal) served with 1 slice plain or toasted wholegrain bread
- 1 × 300g can tomato soup served with 1 slice toasted wholegrain bread; 1 piece fruit
- Prawn Noodle Soup (see recipe, page 164) served with 1 slice wholegrain bread; 1 piece fruit

Dinners

Approx. 400 kcal each. Select one per day.

MEAT DINNERS

- 3 low-fat sausages, grilled, served with 175g (6oz) boiled new potatoes (with skins) and unlimited other vegetables; 1 low-fat yogurt (max. 100 kcal)
- 115g (4oz) any lean meat (beef, lamb, pork), grilled, roasted or dry-fried, served with 115g (4oz) boiled new potatoes (with skins), unlimited other vegetables and low-fat gravy; 1 piece fruit
- 175g (6oz) lamb's liver braised with onions in low-fat gravy and served with 115g (4oz) boiled new potatoes (with skins) and unlimited other vegetables
- 1 × 300g Sainsbury's Cottage Pie served with unlimited vegetables (excluding potatoes)
- Griddled Beef with Provençal Vegetables (see recipe, page 170) served with 115g (4oz) boiled new potatoes (with skins); 1 pear
- Beef and Potato Goulash (see recipe, page 171) served with unlimited vegetables (excluding potatoes); 1 piece fruit
- Fillet Steak with Redcurrant and Thyme Glaze (see recipe, page 175) served with 150g (5oz) boiled new potatoes (with skins) and unlimited other vegetables
- Lemon and Honey Glazed Pork Steaks (see recipe, page 181) served with 115g (4oz) boiled new potatoes (with skins) and unlimited vegetables

continued

- 175g (6oz) lean pork steak, grilled or dry-fried, served with Garlic and Herb Roasted Potatoes (see recipe, page 249) and unlimited other vegetables; 1 piece fruit
- Sweet Chilli Pork (see recipe, page 178) served with 100g (3½oz) boiled new potatoes (with skins) and unlimited green vegetables
- Pork and Pineapple Kebabs (see recipe, page 179) served with 100g (3½oz) boiled new potatoes (with skins), a small mixed salad and 2 tsps sweet chilli sauce
- Fruity pork burgers: mix 115g (4oz) lean minced pork with finely chopped onion, grated apple and chopped sage, then shape into burgers and grill for 6 minutes each side. Serve in 1 × 50g (2oz) wholegrain bap, with 1 tsp mustard plus unlimited salad
- Pastrami Hotpot (see recipe, page 176) served with 1 wholegrain roll
- 1 × 150g (5oz) lean gammon steak, grilled, topped with 1 canned pineapple ring and served with 115g (4oz) boiled new potatoes (with skins) and unlimited green vegetables

CHICKEN AND TURKEY DINNERS

- 1 × 200g (7oz) grilled or baked chicken portion served with 100g (3½oz) boiled new potatoes (with skins) and unlimited other vegetables
- Chicken stir-fry (serves 1): chop 175g (6oz) skinned and boned chicken breast and dry-fry with plenty of freshly ground black pepper in a preheated non-stick pan or wok until almost cooked. Add ½ chopped onion, 3 chopped mushrooms, 1 chopped celery stick, ½ coarsely chopped red or green pepper and cook lightly. Add 2 tbsps soy sauce and toss all the ingredients together. Serve with 1 × 175g (6oz) can beansprouts (place cooked rice and beansprouts into a colander and pour boiling water over to heat through)
- Chicken curry (serves 4): chop 4 × 115g (4 × 4oz) skinned and boned chicken breasts and dry-fry in a preheated non-stick pan. Add 1 large chopped onion and cook until soft. Add 1 × 450g jar any low-fat Indian curry sauce with crispy vegetables, cover and simmer for 15 minutes. Serve with 50g (2oz) [uncooked weight] boiled basmati rice per person
- Japanese chicken kebabs: 1 × 150g (5oz) skinned and boned chicken breast, cut into chunks, marinated in 1 tbsp Japanese soy sauce, 1 tsp mirin, crushed garlic and grated root ginger, then threaded on skewers with red onion quarters and pepper pieces. Grill for 10–15 minutes until cooked and serve with 100g (3½oz) [cooked weight] boiled basmati rice

continued

- Chinese-Style Chicken (see recipe, page 193) served with 50g (2oz) [uncooked weight] boiled basmati rice and unlimited vegetables
- Marinated Barbecue Chicken (see recipe, page 194) served with 100g (3½oz) boiled new potatoes (with skins) and a mixed salad
- Cajun Turkey with Cherry Tomato and Roasted Pepper Salad (see recipe, page 200) served with 115g (4oz) boiled new potatoes (with skins) and a green salad
- Caribbean Chicken Skewers with Mango Salsa (see recipe, page 192) served with 100g (3½oz) boiled new potatoes (with skins) and a green salad
- 1 × 150g (5oz) skinless chicken breast, grilled, served with Sweet and Sour Cucumber (see recipe, page 258) and 50g (2oz) [uncooked weight] boiled basmati rice
- Chicken with Lime and Ginger (see recipe, page 191) served with 115g (4oz) boiled new potatoes (with skins) and unlimited vegetables
- Chicken with Tangerine and Cinnamon (see recipe, page 190) served with 115g (4oz) boiled new potatoes (with skins) and unlimited vegetables
- Any branded low-fat pasta ready meal with chicken or turkey (max. 350 kcal) served with unlimited vegetables (excluding potatoes)

FISH AND SEAFOOD DINNERS

- 175g (6oz) any white fish, grilled, baked or microwaved, served with 175g (6oz) boiled new potatoes (with skins) and unlimited other vegetables plus 1 tbsp low-fat sauce of your choice; 1 low-fat yogurt (max. 100 kcal)
- 1 × 150g (5oz) cod steak, grilled, served with unlimited vegetables (excluding potatoes) and bean purée (made by blending 100g (3½oz) cooked haricot beans with a garlic clove, fresh parsley, lemon juice and 2 tbsps low-fat natural yogurt)
- Marinated Griddled Tuna (see recipe, page 208) served with 115g (4oz) boiled new potatoes (with skins) and 150g (5oz) other vegetables
- 1 × 115g (4oz) fresh salmon steak, grilled, served with 115g (4oz) boiled new potatoes (with skins) and a salad of chicory leaves, cooked green beans and grilled cherry tomatoes all tossed in oil-free dressing
- 1 × 100g (3½oz) fresh salmon steak, grilled, served with Roasted Red Pepper Couscous (see recipe, page 245) and a green salad; 1 piece fresh fruit
- Fresh Salmon Pasta Salad (see recipe, page 210) served with a crisp green salad
- Creamy Grilled Lobster (see recipe, page 211) served with 115g (4oz) boiled new potatoes (with skins) and a green salad
- Seafood Pizza (see recipe, page 212) served with a small salad

continued

- Prawn-Fried Rice (see recipe, page 216) served with a mixed salad; 1 low-fat yogurt (max. 100 kcal)
- Baked Cod with Parma Ham and Saffron Couscous (see recipe, page 204) served with a mixed salad
- Prawn and Mushroom Pasta (see recipe, page 215) served with a mixed salad; 1 piece fruit
- Thai Fish Cakes with Dill Sauce (see recipe, page 203) served with unlimited mixed vegetables or salad
- Spiced Tomato Baked Cod (see recipe, page 202) served with 150g (5oz) boiled new potatoes (with skins) and seasonal vegetables or salad
- Any branded low-fat pasta with fish/seafood ready meal (max. 350 kcal) served with a mixed salad

Remember, you can find more meal suggestions in my original *Gi Jeans Diet*.

VEGETARIAN DINNERS

- Ⓥ 4 Quorn sausages, grilled, and served with 175g (6oz) boiled new potatoes (with skins) or mashed sweet potatoes, and unlimited other vegetables
- Ⓥ 1 Quorn peppered steak, grilled, and served with Ratatouille Mushrooms (see recipe, page 248), 50g (2oz) boiled new potatoes (with skins) and a green salad
- Ⓥ Quorn stir-fry (serves 1): dry-fry 225g (8oz) Quorn chunks with plenty of freshly ground black pepper in a preheated non-stick pan or wok until almost cooked. Add ½ chopped onion, 3 chopped mushrooms, 1 chopped celery stick, ½ coarsely chopped red or green pepper and cook lightly. Add 2 tbsps soy sauce and toss all the ingredients. Serve with 40g (1½oz) [uncooked weight] boiled basmati rice mixed with 1 × 175g (6oz) can beansprouts (place cooked rice and beansprouts into a colander and pour boiling water over to heat through)
- Ⓥ Spicy Quorn noodles: dry-fry 175g (6oz) Quorn mince with chopped red chilli, chopped spring onions and grated root ginger for 3 minutes, then stir in 2 tsps Thai fish sauce, a squeeze of lime juice and 50g (2oz) [uncooked weight] rice noodles. Stir-fry for 2 minutes and serve with sweet chilli sauce and Tomato, Spinach and Balsamic Onion Salad (see recipe, page 260)
- Ⓥ Baked Cheesy Sweet Potatoes (see recipe, page 230) served with a large salad; 1 piece fruit

continued

- Ⓥ Cider and Leek Macaroni Cheese (see recipe, page 227) served with a mixed salad
- Ⓥ 2-egg omelette cooked (without fat) with chopped peppers, onion, mushrooms, peas, tomatoes and herbs and plenty of freshly ground black pepper, and served with 175g (6oz) boiled new potatoes (with skins) or 1 slice wholegrain bread
- Ⓥ Sweet Potato, Pepper and Fennel Bake (see recipe, page 239) served with unlimited vegetables (excluding potatoes) or salad
- Ⓥ Aubergine and Mango Kashmiri (see recipe, page 226) served with 50g (2oz) [uncooked weight] boiled basmati rice
- Ⓥ Vegetarian Chilli (see recipe, page 228) served with Oven-Baked Nachos (see recipe, page 245) and unlimited salad
- Ⓥ Fresh Tomato and Basil Pasta (see recipe, page 232) served with unlimited salad
- Ⓥ Penne with Roasted Vegetables (see recipe, page 223) served with unlimited salad
- Ⓥ Moroccan Chickpeas with Spinach (see recipe, page 219) served with 115g (4oz) boiled new potatoes (with skins) and unlimited other vegetables
- Ⓥ Spinach and Leek Pie (see recipe, page 224) served with 115g (4oz) boiled new potatoes (with skins) and a tomato and mixed leaf salad
- Ⓥ Aubergine and Spinach Pasta Bake (see recipe, page 243) served with a crunchy green salad; 1 piece fruit

continued

- Ⓥ Vegetable Quiche (see recipe, page 229) served with a large salad; 1 × 110g Rosemary Conley Low Fat Belgian Chocolate Mousse
- Ⓥ Any branded low-fat vegetarian ready meal (max. 350 kcal) served with unlimited vegetables (excluding potatoes)

11 The Ultimate Gi Jeans Diet: Part 2

If you have managed to stick strictly to the Ultimate Gi Jeans Kick-start Diet you have done well. Unless you are over 60 years old you can now enjoy more food as well as a daily alcoholic drink (two for men). In addition to this you can still have two Power Snacks each day plus a daily treat that is free of the Gi and low-fat guidelines. That means it can be high in Gi and high in fat so that you never feel forbidden from eating your favourite foods. If you want to eat a bar of chocolate or bag of crisps, you can. Just make sure that you have the equivalent number of calories saved up within your daily allowance.

Part 2 of the Gi Jeans Diet is based on 1500 calories a day of low-fat, low- or medium-Gi foods. For most people who are overweight this is the average optimum calorie allowance to effect a healthy rate of weight loss while giving you plenty to eat and the freedom to have a drink and a treat each day. If you follow the diet strictly and combine it with regular exercise, you should lose 2–2½lb or 1 kilo of body fat each week. Those who are significantly overweight can eat more calories and still achieve this rate of weight loss. For those who have only a few pounds to lose you may find progress slower as your calorie expenditure will obviously be less because there is less of you.

The ideal is to eat the number of calories equal to your basal metabolic rate (BMR), so remember to check the BMR tables on pages 348–51 to find out your personal calorie allowance. If your daily allowance is greater than 1500, you can increase your portion sizes accordingly, for instance by increasing your portion of rice, pasta or potatoes or by having an extra Power Snack or piece of fruit each day. As you lose weight you can adjust your calorie allowance to ensure that your rate of weight loss is maintained (see page 311).

If you have a lot of weight to lose, please be cautious about cutting back on the calories too soon as this could make reaching your ultimate goal much harder. It is in your short- and long-term interests to keep your metabolic rate buoyant. Eating the optimum number of calories to meet your basic metabolic needs is by far the best way to achieve results.

As we get older our metabolic rate slows down so we need fewer daily calories. If we don't reduce the calories as we get older, we can gain weight very easily without realising we are eating too many calories. If you are aged over 60, you may find it easier to stick with the Ultimate Gi Jeans Kick-start Diet, which is based on 1200 calories a day. Alternatively, you could still follow Part 2 of the diet but exclude the alcohol allowance and the treat. Because all the meals and snacks are calorie counted it is simple to make your own selections or substitutions. Depending on your daily calorie allowance you can choose whether or not to eat a dessert after your evening meal.

If you are a solo dieter, take a look at chapter 12, and if you work shifts look at page 145.

So, just follow the rules, select foods you enjoy and wait for the results.

What to do

Each day you can have:

450ml (¾ pint) skimmed or semi-skimmed milk	200 kcal
Breakfast	200 kcal
Lunch	300 kcal
Dinner	500 kcal
2 Power Snacks (50 kcal each)	100 kcal
1 Treat	100 kcal
1 Alcoholic drink*	100 kcal
	Total 1500 kcal

* 2 alcoholic drinks for men

'Free' calories
- Tea and coffee (drunk black or with milk from allowance)
- Water
- Sugar-free soft drinks
- Chopped raw vegetables: cucumber, peppers, carrots, onions, mushrooms, celery and courgettes
- You may take a multi-vitamin supplement each day if you wish
- Depending on your calorie allowance, you can choose whether or not to eat a dessert after your evening meal

Diet notes

Low fat

The term 'low fat' refers to any product with five per cent or less fat.

Bread

Bread should be stoneground or wholegrain (max. 125 calories per slice). Some brands have more than five per cent fat and these are acceptable on this Ultimate Gi Jeans Diet because of their nutritional qualities. For ease of reference, one slice should contain no more than 125 calories.

Breakfast cereals

Choose whole-oat or high-fibre varieties, e.g. All-Bran, Fruit 'n Fibre, Bran Buds, Grapenuts, muesli, Shredded Wheat. Special K is also low Gi, and Weetabix is a natural low-fat, low-sugar option.

Salad

'Salad' includes all salad leaves, cress, tomatoes, cucumber, and chopped raw vegetables such as carrots, peppers, onions, mush-rooms, celery and courgettes. You may serve it with 2 tsps fat-free, low-calorie dressing.

Fruit and vegetables

'1 piece fruit' means one apple, one kiwi, etc., or 115g (4oz) fruit such as strawberries, etc. For the purposes of this diet, one banana counts as two pieces. Choose under-ripe rather than over-ripe ones for a lower Gi rating. For good health, aim to incorporate at least five portions a day of fruit and/or vegetables in your menu selections. Where stated, you are allowed unlimited vegetables with your main course providing they are cooked and served without fat.

Milk

Milk can be skimmed or semi-skimmed, cow's, goat's or soya milk. If 450ml (¾ pint) is too much, you can substitute a low-fat yogurt in place of 150ml (¼ pint) milk. This can be eaten as a dessert or as a between-meal snack.

Drinks

Drink plenty of water, at least five large glasses a day. Tea and coffee may be drunk freely using milk from your allowance. You may also drink unlimited low-calorie soft drinks.

Alcohol

Women may have 100 calories of alcohol per day and men 200 calories. You can save up your allowance for a special occasion if you wish.

Sugar

If you prefer to have more sugar on your breakfast cereal than is included in the diet plan, use a granulated low-calorie alternative.

Rosemary Conley products

At Rosemary Conley we are developing a range of healthy low-fat, low-Gi foods that will be available in several supermarkets. Rosemary Conley low-fat mousses are currently sold in Asda, Waitrose, Morrisons, Co-op and others. My Low Gi Nutrition Bars are sold in Tesco and may be available in other supermarkets. The range is constantly being updated, with new products in development. For information on new products and where they can be purchased, visit the Rosemary Conley website:

www.rosemary-conley.co.uk

Handy portion sizes

If your BMR is higher than 1500, here are some simple suggestions for increasing the calories.

Approx. 50 calories
1 Weetabix or Shredded Wheat
50g (2oz) baked beans
2 grilled turkey rashers
150ml (¼ pint) unsweetened fruit juice
10 grapes

Approx. 100 calories
100g (3½oz) [cooked weight] rice or pasta
115g (4oz) new potatoes
1 slice wholegrain bread
1 large banana
1 large egg (poached, boiled or dry-fried)
1 large low-fat sausage (pork or beef)

Breakfasts

Approx. 200 kcal each. Select one per day.

CEREAL BREAKFASTS

- Ⓥ Any cereal breakfast from the Ultimate Gi Jeans Kick-start Diet menu
- Ⓥ 40g (1½oz) any whole-oat or high-fibre cereal served with milk from allowance and 2 tsps sugar
- Ⓥ 40g (1½oz) any whole-oat or high-fibre cereal (except muesli) served with milk from allowance and topped with 1 chopped banana
- Ⓥ 1 Weetabix served with milk from allowance and 1 tsp sugar, plus 1 banana
- Ⓥ 50g (2oz) All-Bran served with milk from allowance, topped with 115g (4oz) strawberries and 1 tsp sugar
- Ⓥ 50g (2oz) Special K cereal served with milk from allowance and 1 tsp sugar
- Ⓥ 2 Shredded Wheat sprinkled with 1 grated apple and served with milk from allowance and 1 tsp sugar
- Ⓥ 40g (1½ oz) unsweetened muesli mixed with 75g (3oz) 0% fat Greek-style yogurt (e.g. Total 0%) plus 75ml (3fl oz) milk from allowance and low-calorie sweetener to taste

Ⓥ means suitable for vegetarians or vegetarian option is available.

FRUIT BREAKFASTS

- ⓥ Any fruit breakfast from the Ultimate Gi Jeans Kick-start Diet menu
- ⓥ 1 medium banana and 175g (6oz) strawberries or raspberries, sliced, and stirred into 1 × 100g pot low-fat yogurt (max. 75 kcal)
- ⓥ 1 × 213g can prunes in natural juice served with 1 tbsp low-fat yogurt
- ⓥ 225g (8oz) mixed fresh fruit (e.g. chopped melon, raspberries, etc.) topped with 1 × 150g pot 0% fat Greek-style yogurt (e.g. Total 0%)
- ⓥ 115g (4oz) blueberries mixed with 1 pot low-fat yogurt (max. 150 kcal)
- ⓥ Summer Fruit Smoothie (see recipe, page 264), plus 1 banana
- ⓥ Summer Berry Smoothie (see recipe, page 264), plus 1 slice toasted wholegrain bread spread with 1 tsp marmalade
- ⓥ 1 small bottle fruit smoothie (e.g. Innocent Mangoes & Passion Fruit), plus 1 × 35g Rosemary Conley Low Gi Nutrition Bar
- ⓥ 1 medium banana, split lengthways, and topped with 115g (4oz) raspberries and 2 tbsps low-fat yogurt or fromage frais (any flavour)
- ⓥ 1 × 150g probiotic low-fat apricot yogurt, plus 4 chopped dried apricots

COOKED BREAKFASTS

- Ⓥ Any cooked breakfast from the Ultimate Gi Jeans Kick-start Diet menu
- 3 medium low-fat sausages, grilled, served with 150g (5oz) tomatoes (grilled tomatoes or canned tomatoes boiled and reduced to a creamy consistency) and 150g (5oz) grilled mushrooms
- 2 turkey rashers, grilled, served with 2 large grilled tomatoes, 115g (4oz) grilled mushrooms and 50g (2oz) dry-fried sliced onions plus 1 slice toasted wholegrain bread
- ½ bagel, toasted, topped with 3 grilled turkey rashers and 75g (3oz) dry-fried sliced mushrooms
- Ⓥ 2 toasted crumpets spread with 2 tsps marmalade, honey or jam and topped with 1 tbsp 0% fat Greek-style yogurt (e.g. Total 0%)
- 1 medium-sized egg, poached or boiled, served with 2 grilled turkey rashers, unlimited grilled tomatoes and ½ slice toasted wholegrain bread

Lunches

Approx. 300 kcal each. Select one per day.

SANDWICHES, ROLLS AND WRAPS

- BLT: 1 small wholegrain roll spread with reduced-oil salad dressing and filled with 50g (2oz) grilled lean bacon, plus sliced tomato and lettuce; 1 piece fruit
- 2 slices wholegrain bread spread with 2 tsps horseradish sauce and topped with 50g (2oz) pastrami and 4 cherry tomatoes
- 1 small wholegrain roll spread with reduced-oil salad dressing, filled with salad and 75g (3oz) wafer thin ham/chicken/beef/turkey, and served with Crunchy Green Gi Salad (see recipe, page 258)
- 2 slices wholegrain bread spread with low-fat dressing and filled with salad plus one of the following:
  - ○ 115g (4oz) wafer thin ham/chicken/beef
  - ○ Ⓥ 115g (4oz) low-fat cottage cheese
  - ○ 75g (3oz) tuna canned in brine
  - ○ 75g (3oz) crab meat
  - ○ 50g (2oz) mackerel canned in tomato sauce
- Chilli prawn roll: cut 1 wholegrain roll in half and spread each half with 1 triangle Laughing Cow Extra Light Cheese. Mix 1 tbsp sweet chilli sauce with 2 tbsps cooked, shelled prawns and place on top of each half. Add a few rocket or lettuce leaves and season with freshly ground black pepper; 1 piece fruit

continued

- Prawn cocktail open sandwich: mix 115g (4oz) cooked, shelled prawns with 1 heaped tsp low-fat Marie Rose dressing or 2 tsps low-fat salad dressing and place on top of 1 slice wholegrain bread. Serve as an open sandwich with salad
- Parma ham baguette: cut 1 small wholegrain baguette in half and spread with 50g (2oz) Extra Light Philadelphia. Top with 50g (2oz) Parma ham (all visible fat removed) and fresh basil leaves
- 1 × 50g (2oz) pitta bread filled with 50g (2oz) cooked, sliced chicken breast (no skin), plus green salad, sliced cherry tomatoes and 1 tbsp low-fat guacamole
- 1 × 50g (2oz) pitta bread filled with 115g (4oz) crab meat, chopped spring onions, shredded lettuce, chopped fresh coriander and a squeeze of lemon juice
- Ⓥ Any prepacked low-fat sandwich (max. 300 kcal)

SALAD LUNCHES
- Ⓥ Any salad lunch from the Ultimate Gi Jeans Kick-start Diet menu plus 1 piece fruit
- Ⓥ Rice salad: mix 75g (3oz) [cooked weight] boiled basmati rice with chopped spring onions, diced peppers, 1 tbsp sweetcorn, 1 orange, peeled and segmented, and 2 tbsps low-fat fromage frais; 1 piece fruit
- 115g (4oz) wafer thin chicken, beef or ham served with Tomato, Spinach and Balsamic Onion Salad (see recipe, page 260); 1 low-fat yogurt (max. 75 kcal)

continued

- 115g (4oz) [cooked weight] pasta shapes mixed with 115g (4oz) drained canned tuna in brine, chopped spring onions, cucumber, tomato, 1 tbsp sweetcorn kernels and 2 tbsps low-calorie salad dressing, plus 1 small wholegrain roll
- Ⓥ Cheese and coleslaw salad: mix 115g (4oz) low-fat cottage cheese with 115g (4oz) low-fat coleslaw. Season with plenty of black pepper and serve with baby beetroot, sliced cucumber and cherry tomatoes plus 1 slice wholegrain bread
- 1 × 100g (3½oz) can pink salmon in brine, drained, mixed with salad leaves, sliced peppers, cucumber chunks, spring onions and cherry tomatoes all tossed in oil-free dressing and served with 1 small wholegrain roll; 1 peach or nectarine
- Prawn salad: mix 115g (4oz) cooked, shelled prawns with 115g (4oz) [cooked weight] pasta shells, 1 tbsp low-fat Marie Rose dressing, 1 tbsp low-fat yogurt and freshly ground black pepper. Serve with Crunchy Green Gi Salad (see recipe, page 258)
- 50g (2oz) smoked mackerel served with Sweet Potato and Cucumber Salad (see recipe, page 259)
- 50g (2oz) smoked mackerel or 75g (3oz) fresh salmon served with 75g (3oz) boiled new potatoes (with skins) and a small salad
- Orange and Fennel Greek Salad (see recipe, page 261) served with 1 wholegrain roll; 1 low-fat yogurt (max. 75 kcal)
- Ⓥ Any prepacked low-fat salad (max. 300 kcal)

SOUP LUNCHES

- ⓥ 1 × 400g can any branded lentil or vegetable soup (max. 200 kcal) served with 1 slice wholegrain bread or a small wholegrain roll
- ⓥ Gazpacho: blend 200g (7oz) skinned tomatoes, 1 garlic clove, ¼ peeled cucumber and 1 tsp white wine vinegar until smooth. Garnish with diced peppers, red onion, and cucumbers and chill. Serve with 1 small wholegrain roll; 1 apple, pear or orange
- ⓥ Chilli Bean Soup (see recipe, page 162) served with 1 slice wholegrain bread
- ⓥ Carrot and Parsnip Soup (see recipe, page 166) served with 1 slice wholegrain bread
- ⓥ Roast Pepper Gazpacho (see recipe, page 163) served with 1 slice wholegrain bread; 1 low-fat yogurt (max. 100 kcal)
- Thai Chicken Soup (see recipe, page 165); 1 banana
- Seafood Chowder (see recipe, page 168) served with 1 small wholegrain roll

COOKED LUNCHES

- ⓥ Any cooked lunch from the Ultimate Gi Jeans Kick-start Diet menu plus 1 piece fruit
- 1 × 175g (6oz) sweet potato baked in its skin, topped with 115g (4oz) canned tuna in brine and 25g (1oz) sweetcorn mixed with 1 tbsp chopped chives and 4 tsps low-calorie salad dressing

continued

- 1 × 200g (7oz) sweet potato baked in its skin, topped with Arrabbiata Prawns (see recipe, page 214) and served with unlimited salad; 1 low-fat yogurt (max. 100 kcal)
- Ⓥ 1 × 175g (6oz) sweet potato baked in its skin, topped with 4 tbsps baked beans, and served with a large salad
- 2 low-fat sausages, grilled, served with 115g (4oz) baked beans, 10 grilled cherry tomatoes, 115g (4oz) grilled mushrooms and ½ slice toasted wholegrain bread
- Chicken tikka kebabs: cut 115g (4oz) skinned and boned chicken breast into chunks and mix with 1 tbsp chicken tikka sauce. Cook under a hot grill for 10–15 minutes, turning halfway through. Serve with Minted Cumber and Onion Salad (see recipe, page 256) and 1 mini pitta bread
- Ⓥ 1 × 115g (4oz) salmon fillet, chargrilled, steamed or poached, served with cooked asparagus drizzled with lemon juice and scattered with black pepper and chilli flakes, plus 100g (3½oz) boiled new potatoes (with skins)
- Ⓥ Omelette made with 2 eggs: cook eggs in a non-stick frying pan with a little spray oil (e.g. Fry Light), 75g (3oz) chopped mixed peppers and ½ red onion. Just before folding and serving add some chopped fresh herbs; 1 piece fresh fruit
- 1 slice toasted wholegrain bread topped with 50g (2oz) sardines in tomato sauce; Kiwi and Mango Salad with Lime Maple Syrup (see recipe, page 265)

continued

- Ⓥ Garlic Mushrooms (see recipe, page 254) served with 1 slice wholegrain bread and a large green salad
- Ⓥ 2 Roasted Mediterranean Tartlets (see recipe, page 220) served with salad; 1 piece fruit
- Ⓥ Vegetable stir-fry: dissolve a vegetable stock cube in a pan of boiling water. Add 50g (2oz) [uncooked weight] basmati rice and cook for 10 minutes. Preheat a non-stick frying pan or wok and sprinkle with freshly ground black pepper. Add a selection of chopped vegetables, e.g. onions, peppers, mushrooms, celery, courgettes, chilli. Stir frequently and, when almost cooked, add half a sachet of Blue Dragon stir-fry sauce of your choice. Drain the rice and serve with the vegetable stir-fry
- 100g (3½oz) low-fat tandoori chicken fillets, cooked, served with Fried Carrots and Green Chillies (see recipe, page 255) and raita (3 tbsps natural yogurt mixed with 1 tsp mint sauce and chopped cucumber); 1 piece fruit
- Ⓥ Tofu Noodle Stir-fry (see recipe, page 242)
- Ⓥ Pasta in tomato and basil sauce: cook 100g (3½oz) [uncooked weight] penne pasta in boiling water with a vegetable stock cube. Drain and return to the pan. Add a small jar of tomato and basil cook-in-sauce and more fresh basil to taste
- Ⓥ Spaghetti Napoletana: dry-fry ½ chopped onion, 1 diced red pepper and 1 crushed garlic clove for 5 minutes. Add 1 small can chopped tomatoes and heat through. Serve with 50g (2oz) [uncooked weight] boiled spaghetti and a sprinkling of Parmesan

continued

- Turkey and Pepper Burgers (see recipe, page 198) served with 115g (4oz) boiled new potatoes (with skins) and a large salad

QUICK AND EASY LUNCHES

- Ⓥ 1 slice toasted wholegrain bread topped with 1 × 200g can baked beans and served with a large salad
- 50g (2oz) smoked mackerel fillet served with 1 tsp horseradish sauce and a large mixed salad, plus 1 slice wholegrain bread
- Ⓥ Goat's cheese toastie: 2 slices toasted wholegrain bread rubbed with fresh garlic and covered with chopped cherry tomatoes, red onion and fresh herbs. Top with 1 × 15g (½oz) slice goat's cheese, and grill
- 115g (4oz) cooked chicken breast (no skin) served with a large mixed salad, plus 1 small wholegrain roll
- Sardines on toast: 1 slice toasted wholegrain bread topped with 100g (3½oz) sardines in tomato sauce. Sprinkle with balsamic vinegar and a little chopped basil. Place under a hot grill and heat through; 1 piece fruit
- Mix together 1 chopped green pepper, 1 chopped tomato, chopped cucumber, 50g (2oz) [uncooked weight] boiled basmati rice, 25g (1oz) peas and 25g (1oz) sweetcorn. Add soy sauce and black pepper to taste and serve with 50g (2oz) wafer thin ham or beef
- Ⓥ 1 × 200g can baked beans (eaten cold); 1 × 35g Rosemary Conley Low Gi Nutrition Bar plus 1 kiwi fruit

Dinners

Approx. 500 kcal each. Select one per day.

Where the calories allow, a dessert has been included in these dinner menus. You can substitute a dessert of your choice, providing you do not exceed the calories available. Where no dessert has been included you can use the 100 calories available from your treat or alcohol allowance if you wish.

In addition to the following menus, you may also choose any item from the Ultimate Gi Jeans Kick-start Diet dinner menu and have it with a dessert from the list on page 136 or with an extra glass of wine. You can also find more dinner options in my original *Gi Jeans Diet*.

BEEF DINNERS

- 115g (4oz) lean fillet or rump steak, grilled, served with 115g (4oz) boiled new potatoes (with skins), unlimited green vegetables, grilled tomatoes and mushrooms; 1 Rosemary Conley Low Fat Belgian Chocolate Mousse or 1 low-fat yogurt or fromage frais (max. 125 kcal)
- Roast Beef with Yorkshire Pudding and Dry-roast Sweet Potatoes (see recipe, page 172) served with unlimited other vegetables
- Beef Masala (see recipe, page 174) served with 50g (2oz) [uncooked weight] boiled basmati rice
- Creamy Madeira Beef (see recipe, page 169) served with 175g (6oz) mashed sweet potatoes creamed with virtually fat-free fromage frais and unlimited other vegetables
- Beef and vegetable bolognese: dry-fry 75g (3oz) extra lean minced beef in a non-stick pan or wok until browned. Add 1 small chopped onion, 1 crushed garlic clove, 1 finely sliced carrot and 225g (8oz) sliced mushrooms. Cook for 5 minutes, then add 1 × 200g can tomatoes, a pinch of mixed herbs, 1 crumbled beef stock cube and a splash of red wine. Season to taste with freshly ground black pepper. Bring to the boil and simmer gently until the vegetables are cooked and the sauce has thickened. Serve with 50g (2oz) [uncooked weight] boiled spaghetti and a large salad; 225g (8oz) fresh fruit salad

LAMB DINNERS

- 115g (4oz) lamb steak, grilled, served with 115g (4oz) boiled new potatoes (with skins), unlimited other vegetables, mint sauce and low-fat gravy; 1 low-fat yogurt (max. 150 kcal)

- Chilli lamb: mix together 1 tbsp chilli sauce, with ½ tbsp each plum sauce, tomato ketchup and water. Place 1 lean lamb steak under a preheated grill for 4–6 minutes each side, turning once. Halfway through cooking the second side, brush the steak with sauce and continue cooking for the final 2–3 minutes. Serve with 50g (2oz) [uncooked weight] boiled basmati rice or pasta, any remaining sauce and a mixed salad; 1 piece fruit

- Italian Shepherd's Pie (see recipe, page 182) served with unlimited vegetables; Melon Sunrise (see recipe, page 269)

- Lamb Chasseur (see recipe, page 183) served with 150g (5oz) boiled new potatoes (with skins) and unlimited vegetables; 1 piece fruit

PORK AND GAMMON DINNERS

- 1 × 115g (4oz) lean pork steak, grilled, served with apple sauce, 1 tbsp sage and onion stuffing (made from a packet with water), 115g (4oz) boiled new potatoes (with skins) and unlimited other vegetables; 1 piece fruit
- 1 × 175g (6oz) lean pork fillet, sprinkled with soy sauce, then grilled or dry-fried, and served with 50g (2oz) [uncooked weight] boiled noodles and Stir-Fried Mushroom and Peppers (see recipe, page 250)
- 2 large low-fat pork sausages, grilled, served with 115g (4oz) boiled new potatoes (with skins) and unlimited other vegetables; Rosemary Conley Low Fat Mousse, any flavour
- 4 medium low-fat pork sausages, grilled, served with 115g (4oz) boiled new or sweet potatoes, mashed with milk or yogurt and seasoned well, plus 1 × 200g can baked beans and 10 grilled cherry tomatoes
- Spicy Meatballs with Spaghetti (see recipe, page 180) served with Crunchy Green Gi Salad (see recipe, page 258)
- 1 × 150g (5oz) lean gammon steak, grilled, served with 1 tbsp apple sauce, 115g (4oz) boiled new potatoes (with skins) and unlimited green vegetables; 1 low-fat yogurt (max. 100 kcal)
- Quick Sausage Casserole (see recipe, page 177) served with 115g (4oz) boiled new potatoes (with skins) and unlimited vegetables; Mango and Whisky Mousse (see recipe, page 267)

CHICKEN AND TURKEY DINNERS

- 1 × 115g (4oz) skinned chicken breast, grilled or oven-baked in foil with 1 tsp mango chutney, served with chargrilled vegetables (cherry tomatoes, slices of courgettes, chunks of red and green pepper and quarters of red onion) plus 50g (2oz) [uncooked weight] boiled basmati rice and soy sauce; Kiwi and Mango Salad with Lime Maple Syrup (see recipe, page 265)

- 175g (6oz) skinned chicken breast, grilled or oven-baked in foil, served with Roast Sweet Potatoes with Chilli Glaze (see recipe, page 247) and unlimited green vegetables

- Chicken kebabs: cut 150g (5oz) skinned and boned chicken breast into chunks and thread on a skewer with green peppers and cherry tomatoes. Brush with soy sauce and place under a hot grill until the chicken is cooked. Serve with 1 tsp satay sauce and 50g (2oz) [uncooked weight] boiled basmati rice or pasta

- Garlicky Chicken Kiev (see recipe, page 187) served with 150g (5oz) boiled new potatoes (with skins) and unlimited other vegetables

- Cheesy Bacon Chicken (see recipe, page 188) served with 50g (2oz) [uncooked weight] boiled noodles and green salad

- Spicy Chicken Pasta (see recipe, page 195) served with unlimited salad; 1 piece fruit

- Tomato, Chicken and Ginger Stir-Fry (see recipe, page 186) served with 50g (2oz) [uncooked weight] boiled basmati rice

continued

- 175g (6oz) chicken pieces, stir-fried with chopped onion, peppers, mushrooms, courgettes and sweetcorn plus ½ can low-fat wine cook-in-sauce, and served with 50g (2oz) [uncooked weight] boiled basmati rice
- Chicken stir-fry: cut 115g (4oz) skinned and boned chicken breast into strips and dry-fry in a hot non-stick frying pan with plenty of black pepper. When almost cooked, add 1 small crushed garlic clove, 115g (4oz) chopped fresh vegetables (e.g. courgettes, celery, onion, green, red, yellow peppers, mangetout, carrots and beansprouts). Add a little grated fresh root ginger. Stir in ½ packet any Blue Dragon stir-fry sauce until the chicken and vegetables are well coated and serve immediately with 50g (2oz) [uncooked weight] boiled basmati rice
- Green Thai Chicken Curry (see recipe, page 189) served with 50g (2oz) [uncooked weight] boiled basmati rice and unlimited salad tossed in oil-free dressing
- Spicy Lemon Chicken (see recipe, page 185) served with 50g (2oz) [uncooked weight] boiled basmati rice; 1 piece fruit
- Chicken and Spinach Lasagne (see recipe, page 196) served with Crunchy Green Gi Salad (see recipe, page 258)
- Turkey Amatriciana (see recipe, page 199) served with Crunchy Green Gi Salad (see recipe, page 258)

FISH AND SEAFOOD DINNERS

- 225g (8oz) any white fish, grilled, steamed or microwaved, served with 115g (4oz) boiled new potatoes (with skins) and unlimited other vegetables plus parsley sauce made with skimmed milk; 1 × 110g Rosemary Conley Low Fat Belgian Chocolate Mousse
- 1 × 175g (6oz) salmon steak, grilled, served with 115g (4oz) boiled new potatoes (with skins) and unlimited other vegetables
- 150g (5oz) fresh salmon, marinated in teriyaki sauce, then grilled, and served with 115g (4oz) boiled new potatoes (with skins) and unlimited green vegetables or salad; 200g (7oz) fresh fruit salad
- 1 × 200g (7oz) fresh tuna steak, grilled, served with 115g (4oz) boiled new potatoes (with skins) and Griddled Asparagus with Fresh Lemon and Cracked Black Pepper (see recipe, page 251)
- 2 × 115g (2 × 4oz) plaice fillets, sprinkled with lemon juice and chopped fresh herbs, then grilled in foil or steamed, and served with broccoli and sliced courgettes; 1 meringue basket filled with 75g (3oz) fresh fruit and topped with 1 tbsp low-fat yogurt or Rosemary Conley Low Fat Mousse
- Mediterranean Fish Stew (see recipe, page 205) served with 75g (3oz) [uncooked weight] boiled basmati rice
- Baked Salmon with Tomato and Lime Salsa (see recipe, page 206) served with Roasted Red Pepper Couscous (see recipe, page 245)
- Tuna and Sweetcorn Pasta (see recipe, page 209) served with a mixed salad

VEGETARIAN DINNERS

- Ⓥ Cheesy vegetable macaroni: dry-fry unlimited button mushrooms, cherry tomatoes and sliced leeks in a non-stick pan with a little spray oil (e.g. Fry Light). Mix in 115g (4oz) [cooked weight] boiled macaroni and cover with low-fat béchamel sauce made with skimmed milk (e.g. Crosse & Blackwell Béchamel Sauce or Tesco Readymade Fresh White Sauce). Top with 2 tsps low-fat Cheddar cheese and grill until golden brown; 1 piece fruit

- Ⓥ Thai veggie curry: cook chopped spring onions, sliced aubergine, peppers, mangetout, broccoli florets and thin green beans in a non-stick pan with a little spray oil. Add 1 tsp green curry paste and 150ml (¼ pint) low-fat coconut milk and heat through. Serve with fresh coriander and 75g (3oz) [cooked weight] boiled egg noodles; 1 low-fat yogurt (max. 100 kcal)

- Ⓥ Ratatouille with pasta: heat ½ large can ratatouille and serve with 50g (2oz) [uncooked weight] boiled pasta sprinkled with 1 tbsp grated Parmesan cheese, plus a mixed salad; 2 pieces fruit or 1 low-fat yogurt (max. 100 kcal)

- Ⓥ Dry-fry 175g (6oz) Quorn pieces with 1 chopped onion. Pour in ½ can low-fat wine cook-in-sauce and heat gently for 15–20 minutes. Serve with 50g (2oz) [uncooked weight] boiled basmati rice and unlimited green vegetables; 1 × 110g Rosemary Conley Low Fat Belgian Chocolate Mousse

continued

- Ⓥ 4 Quorn sausages, grilled, served with 115g (4oz) boiled new potatoes (with skins), 115g (4oz) peas and unlimited grilled tomatoes; 2 pieces fruit
- Ⓥ 2 Quorn Pork Style Ribsters, grilled, served with 115g (4oz) boiled new potatoes (with skins) and unlimited green vegetables and grilled tomatoes; 2 pieces fruit or 1 low-fat yogurt (max. 100 kcal)
- Ⓥ 1 Quorn Lemon and Pepper Fillet, dry-fried, served with Lentil Salad (see recipe, page 231); 1 piece fruit
- Ⓥ 2 Quorn Lamb Style Grills, grilled, served with Baked Winter Vegetables (see recipe, page 252), 150g (5oz) boiled new potatoes (with skins) and mint sauce
- Ⓥ Vegetable fajitas: wrap chargrilled sliced peppers and red onions in 1 tortilla and top with 1 tbsp very low-fat plain fromage frais and 1 tbsp low-fat guacamole. Serve with unlimited salad and a little salsa
- Ⓥ 1 vegetarian burger, grilled, served with 4 grilled tomatoes, 115g (4oz) grilled mushrooms, 115g (4oz) peas, and 175g (6oz) boiled new potatoes (with skins). Serve with sauce or pickle of your choice; 1 low-fat yogurt (max. 60 kcal)
- Ⓥ Lentil Roast (see recipe, page 238) served with Sautéed Courgettes and Cherry Tomatoes (see recipe, page 253); 1 low-fat yogurt (max. 100 kcal)
- Ⓥ Vegetarian Chilli (see recipe, page 228) served with 50g (2oz) [uncooked weight] boiled basmati rice
- Ⓥ Asparagus and Vegetable Bake (see recipe, page 235) served with a green salad

continued

- Ⓥ Spinach and Ricotta Cannelloni (see recipe, page 236) served with Crunchy Green Gi Salad (see recipe, page 258)
- Ⓥ Parsnip and Chestnut Herb Roast (see recipe, page 233) served with 75g (3oz) Dry-roasted Sweet Potatoes (see recipe, page 172) and unlimited other vegetables
- Ⓥ Mexican Bean Bites with Red Pepper Sauce (see recipe, page 218) served with 100g (3½oz) boiled new potatoes (with skins) and unlimited other vegetables
- Ⓥ Roasted Butternut Squash and Tomato Tart (see recipe, page 234) served with 115g (4oz) boiled new potatoes (with skins) and unlimited other vegetables.
- Ⓥ Spicy Chickpea Burgers (see recipe, page 217) served with salad and 100g (3½oz) low-fat oven chips and 5 grilled cherry tomatoes
- Ⓥ Any low-fat ready meal (max. 450 kcal), plus unlimited mixed salad

Desserts

Depending on your calorie allowance and whether having a dessert is really important to you, in Part 2 of the Ultimate Gi Jeans Diet you can select a dinner suggestion from the Kick-start Diet menus and add one of the following dessert ideas, all with five per cent or less fat. You could also use your 100-calorie alcohol allowance for a dessert, if you wish, or use your treat calories. Remember, for a diet to be successful, it must satisfy your taste buds and personal needs.

100-CALORIE DESSERTS

- 1 meringue nest filled with 1 tbsp low fat yogurt or 0% fat Greek-style yogurt and topped with 50g (2oz) strawberries or raspberries
- 200g (7oz) fresh fruit salad
- 200g (7oz) seedless grapes
- 1 large banana
- 1 yogurt or fromage frais (max. 100 kcal and 5% fat)
- 1 Shape Orange or Lemon Greek-style Yogurt
- 1 pot Rowntrees Low Sugar Jelly (any flavour) topped with 50g (2oz) strawberries and 1 tbsp low-fat yogurt
- 115g (4oz) fresh pineapple with 1 tsp 0% fat Greek-style yogurt (e.g. Total 0%)
- 1 readymade dessert (max. 100 kcal and 5% fat)
- 1 × 110g Rosemary Conley Low Fat Mousse – Belgian Chocolate, Strawberry or Orange
- ½ melon, any type, filled with 50g (2oz) raspberries
- 1 × 35g Rosemary Conley Low Gi Nutrition Bar

- 1 meringue nest filled with 1 tsp Rosemary Conley Low Fat Mousse – Belgian Chocolate Mousse, Strawberry or Orange and 1 sliced strawberry
- Strawberry brûlée: place 100g (3½oz) strawberries in the bottom of a ramekin dish. Top with 85g (3oz) 0% fat Greek-style yogurt (e.g. Total 0%) and 2 tsps demerara sugar. Place under a preheated hot grill until the sugar caramelises
- 115g (4oz) fresh or frozen raspberries served with 1 low-fat raspberry-flavoured yogurt (max. 75 kcal)
- 1 meringue nest filled with 25g (1oz) any fruit and topped with 1 tbsp low-fat fromage frais
- Mango and Whisky Mousse (see recipe, page 267)
- Blueberry Syllabub (see recipe, page 262)
- Fruity Coconut Milk Jelly (see recipe, page 268)
- Banana Bread Pudding (see recipe, page 270)
- Mixed Grape Chill (see recipe, page 269)
- Kiwi and Mango Salad with Lime Maple Syrup (see recipe, page 265)
- Melon Sunrise (see recipe, page 269)
- Raspberry Baked Meringues (see recipe, page 266)
- Compote of Summer Fruits with Vanilla Yogurt (see recipe, page 271)
- Gratin of Pink Grapefruit and Orange (see recipe, page 263)
- Wine-Poached Apricots with Raspberries (see recipe, page 272)
- 1 Ryvita Dark Rye crispbread topped with 25g (1oz) low-fat Cheddar cheese and 1 tsp pickle

Power Snacks

Approx. 50 kcal each. Select two per day.

The following Power Snacks have been chosen because of their low Gi rating. They are slow-releasing energy foods that will help sustain your blood sugar levels until your next meal. Eat one mid-morning and one mid-afternoon.

FRESH FRUIT
- 2 kiwi fruits
- 1 small or ½ large banana
- 1 medium pear
- 1 medium peach
- 1 medium apple
- 1 medium nectarine
- 1 medium orange
- 1 whole papaya
- 2 satsumas
- 2 fresh figs
- 2 clementines
- 3 plums
- 4 apricots
- 100g (3½oz) pineapple
- 75g (3oz) seedless grapes
- 100g (3½oz) mango
- 100g (3½oz) cherries
- 1 whole grapefruit
- 150g (5oz) strawberries or raspberries plus 1 tsp 0% fat Greek-style yogurt (e.g. Total 0%)

DRIED FRUIT

- 2 apricots
- 1 fig
- 20g (¾oz) sultanas

VEGETABLES

- 8 cherry tomatoes
- 150g (5oz) mixed salad with 1 tsp fat-free dressing
- 8 carrot sticks with 25g (1oz) salsa
- 3 celery sticks with 25g (1oz) low-fat cottage cheese mixed with black pepper and chopped red onion
- 200g (7oz) mixed salad
- 200g (7oz) Crunchy Green Gi Salad (see recipe, page 258)

OTHER POWER SNACKS

- 1 Ryvita Dark Rye crispbread spread with 15g (½oz) low-fat humous
- 15g (½oz) toasted muesli served with milk from allowance and a little low-calorie sugar substitute
- 1 × 100g pot 0.1% fat Actimel probiotic yogurt drink, any flavour, plus 1 satsuma or clementine

Treats

Approx. 100 kcal each. Select one per day.

You can choose any food or drink you like for your 100-calorie treat, and it can fall outside the low-fat, low-Gi guidelines. You can also save up your treats for a special occasion. Remember, it is *your* choice and *your* treat. Here are some suggestions.

Treats with more than five per cent fat

SAVOURY TREATS

- 1 mini Babybel Light plus 2 Ryvita Dark Rye crispbreads
- 100g (3½oz) olives (weighed with stones)
- ½ avocado with 1 tsp low-calorie dressing
- 15g (½oz) peanut butter
- 1 × 22g bag Walkers French Fries Salt & Vinegar
- 1 × 23g Walkers Squares Ready Salted
- 1 × 24g bag Kettle Crispy Bakes Mild Cheese with Sweet Onion
- 1 × 21g bag Tayto Advantage Cheddar & Onion Crispy Lites
- 1 × 21g bag Golden Wonder Golden Lights Sour Cream & Onion Flavour
- 1 × 21g bag Boots Shapers Crunchy Salt & Vinegar Sticks
- 10 Pringles Light Sour Cream & Onion
- 1 × 25g bag Jacob's Original Twiglets

NUTTY TREATS

- 15g (½oz) Brazil nuts
- 15g (½oz) pine nuts
- 15g (½oz) walnuts
- 15g (½oz) pecans
- 20g (¾oz) hazelnuts
- 20g (¾oz) almonds
- 20g (¾oz) pistachio nuts
- 20g (¾oz) mixed nuts and raisins

CEREAL BARS

- 1 Boots Shapers Chocolate & Juicy Raisin Cereal Bar
- 1 Kellogg's Special K Chocolate Chip Bar
- 1 Kellogg's All-Bran Honey & Oat Bar
- 1 Slim-Fast Cranberry, Almond & Raisin Snack Bar
- 1 Kellogg's Nutri-Grain Chewy
- 1 Nestlé Honey Nut Cheerios Cereal and Milk Bar
- 1 Seeds of Change Organic Strawberry Cereal Bar
- 1 Tesco Healthy Living Chocolate & Orange Cereal Bar
- 1 Harvest Chewee White Choc Chip Cereal Bar

SWEET TREATS

- 2 slices Terry's Chocolate Orange
- 1 Boots Shapers Double Chocolate Treat
- 1 fun size bag M&Ms
- 1 Cadbury Dairy Milk Under 99 Kcal Bar
- 3 Cadbury Chocolate Fingers
- 4 Nestlé After Eight Straws
- 3 Nestlé After Eight Mints
- 2 Cadbury Crunchie Chunks
- 6 Nestlé Aero Bubbles
- 1 Mr Kipling Chocolate Sponge slice
- 1 McVitie's Milk Chocolate Digestive
- 1 Tunnock's Milk Chocolate Tea Cake
- 1 McVitie's Milk Chocolate Digestive
- 2 McVitie's Jaffa Cakes
- 4 Werther's Originals Butter Candies
- 20 Smarties
- 1 × 20g packet mini Jammie Dodgers
- 1 shortbread finger

Treats with five per cent or less fat

CEREAL BARS

- 1 Waitrose Perfectly Balanced Cereal Bar (Sultana & Honey, Ginger, Apricot, Cranberry)
- 1 Tesco Healthy Living Cranberry & Blackcurrant Bar
- 1 Tesco Healthy Living Maple Cereal Bar
- 1 Asda Good For You Apple & Cinnamon Cereal Bar
- 1 Morrisons Eat Smart Chewy Cranberry Breakfast Bar
- 1 McVitie's Go Ahead Apricot Fruit Tops

SWEET TREATS

- 6 Bassett's Liquorice Allsorts
- 10 Bassett's Milky Babies
- 5 Starburst Sweets
- 1 pot Hartley's Low Sugar Strawberry Jelly plus 1 tbsp 0% fat Greek yogurt
- 100g (3½oz) fresh raspberries with 1 serving Bird's Dream Topping
- 1 pot Tesco Healthy Living Lemon Cheesecake Yogurt
- 1 meringue nest with 50g (2oz) Yeo Valley Organic Raspberry Yogurt
- 1 M&S Count On Us Blueberry & Vanilla Flavour Cookie
- 2 Caxton Pink 'n' Whites Wafers
- 6 M&S Count On Us Chocolate Biscuit Sticks
- 6 Fox's Officially Low Fat Cranberry & Honey Biscuit Fingers

SAVOURY TREATS

- 1 Tesco Healthy Living Dutch Crispbake spread with 30g extra light soft cheese and topped with 1 smoked salmon slice
- 1 × 25g serving Penn State Original Salted Pretzels
- 1 × 25g bag Jacob's Thai Bites
- 1 × 25g bag Sainsbury's Be Good To Yourself Sea Salt & Cracked Black Pepper Pretzel Sticks
- 1 × 25g bag Sainsbury's Be Good To Yourself Sour Cream & Chive Flavour Hoops
- 1 × 25g bag M&S Count On Us Smokey Ham Flavour Bagel Bakes
- 1 × 30g bag Ryvita Minis Sweet Chilli
- 1 × 25g bag M&S Count On Us Pretzel Loops

LIQUID TREATS

- 1 Cadbury Highlights chocolate drink
- 1 × 150ml (5fl oz) glass red or dry white wine or champagne
- 1 double pub measure gin or vodka and slimline tonic
- 1 double pub measure rum and Diet Coke
- 1 double pub measure whisky or cognac
- 300ml (½ pint) beer, lager or dry cider

Sample menu plan
for shift workers

If you work shifts it's best to think of your diet in 'one-week' chunks rather than in days. If your personal daily calorie allowance is 1500, then over a week you should consume 10,500 calories. A shift worker needs to have five meals a day, which will, in effect, include two breakfasts. So, have breakfast before you go to bed and again when you get up (allow an extra 100 calories with one option). Then have two Power Snacks and a main meal plus dessert to suit your shift pattern, and enjoy an alcoholic drink. So over a 24-hour period your menu plan could look like this:

Daily allowance
- 450ml (¾ pint) semi-skimmed milk   200 kcal
- 1 alcoholic drink   100 kcal

BREAKFAST 1 (before bed)
- 3 medium low-fat sausages, grilled, and served
  with 150g (5oz) grilled mushrooms and 150g
  (5oz) canned tomatoes boiled and reduced to
  a creamy consistency)   200 kcal
- 1 slice toasted wholegrain bread   100 kcal

BREAKFAST 2 (on rising)
- 40g (1½oz) unsweetened muesli topped with
  1 chopped apple or pear and served with milk
  from allowance   200 kcal

continued

MAIN MEAL

- Chicken and Spinach Lasagne (see recipe, page 196) served with a green salad   500 kcal
- 115g (4oz) fresh or frozen raspberries served with 1 low-fat raspberry-flavoured yogurt (max. 75 kcal)   100 kcal

POWER SNACKS (2 per day)

- 1 apple   50 kcal
- 2 satsumas   50 kcal

N.B. You can choose which type of breakfast to have before you go to bed and when you get up. It depends on the time of day or night. For instance, if you are going to bed soon after you finish your shift, it's best to go for the cereal option before bed and the cooked option when you get up.

12 The Ultimate Gi Jeans Solo Slim Diet

Trying to lose weight on your own needn't be difficult and with careful planning it can be easier than you think.

Here you will find seven breakfasts, lunches and dinners, as well as additional Power Snacks to see you through each day with minimal shopping requirements while giving you all the nutrients you need for good health.

For the first two weeks of the diet follow the Solo Slim Kickstart Diet by eating one breakfast, one lunch and one dinner each day, plus two Power Snacks, in addition to your milk allowance and try to incorporate five portions of fruit or vegetables into your menu choices each day, as this is important for good health.

After the initial two weeks, you can then move on to the much more generous Part 2 of the diet. As well as your three meals and your two 50-calorie Power Snacks each day, you may also select a 100-calorie treat, an alcoholic drink and a 100-calorie dessert. It is up to you how you use these extra 300 calories, which means that your eating plan will not seem like a diet at all.

This Solo Slim Diet offers you a free-choice menu where you can select any meal to suit your taste buds and lifestyle, although I have designed a seven-day menu planner for the Kick-start Diet to show how this might be done and created a shopping list to help you achieve it. You can move the meals around and duplicate those that you enjoy most of all. Of course, if you make your own substitutions, you will have to amend your shopping list accordingly. For your dessert, alcohol selection and your treats in Part 2 of the diet, you will find suggestions in the main diet section on pages 136–144.

You are allowed 450ml (¾ pint) skimmed or semi-skimmed milk each day to take in your unlimited cups of tea and coffee as well as with your breakfast cereal. Alternatively, you can substitute a low-fat yogurt (max. 75 kcal) for 150ml (¼ pint) milk if you prefer. Remember to amend your shopping list.

Daily calorie allowance

WEEKS 1 AND 2

450ml (¾ pint) milk	200 kcal
Breakfast	200 kcal
Mid-morning Power Snack	50 kcal
Lunch	300 kcal
Mid-afternoon Power Snack	50 kcal
Dinner	400 kcal
TOTAL	1200 kcal

FROM WEEK 3

450ml (¾ pint) milk	200 kcal
Breakfast	200 kcal
Mid-morning Power Snack	50 kcal
Lunch	300 kcal
Mid-afternoon Power Snack	50 kcal
Dinner	400 kcal
Dessert	100 kcal
Treat	100 kcal
Alcohol	100 kcal
TOTAL	1500 kcal

Weekly shopping list

N.B. VEGETARIANS: Vegetarians can replace meat and fish with Quorn products of equivalent calorie values.

Dairy
2.8 litres (5 pints) skimmed or semi-skimmed milk
1 × 150g pot 0% fat Greek-style yogurt (e.g. Total 0%)
6 large eggs
1 × 50g pot low-fat cottage cheese

Bread
2 small sliced wholegrain loaves

Breakfast cereals
Your choice: e.g. porridge oats, Weetabix, muesli

Fresh meat, fish, and chicken

1 × 150g pack turkey rashers

1 pack lean smoked bacon

50g (2oz) wafer thin ham

3 × 150g (3 × 5oz) chicken breasts

1 × 115g (4oz) fresh salmon steak or 1 small can red salmon

175g (6oz) white fish (in place of one chicken portion)

Fresh vegetables

2 large sweet potatoes

300g (11oz) baby new potatoes

400g (14oz) broccoli

6 carrots

1 small cabbage

200g (7oz) French beans

3 peppers (1 green, 1 red, 1 yellow)

115g (4oz) fresh button mushrooms

1 red onion

1 Spanish onion

1 pillow pack mixed salad leaves

1 pack cherry tomatoes

½ cucumber

1 head of celery

Fresh herbs and spices

Chives

1 garlic bulb

Fresh fruit

3 small bananas

1 grapefruit

6 satsumas
350g (12oz) strawberries
4 kiwi fruits
225g (8oz) grapes

Canned or frozen foods
3 small cans tuna in brine
1 × 220g can plum tomatoes
2 × 200g cans chopped tomatoes
1 × 200g can baked beans
2 small cans sweetcorn kernels
1 small can mushrooms in brine (or use fresh mushrooms
    if you prefer – add 25g/1oz to fresh quantity)
1 × 350g jar sweet and sour stir-fry sauce
1 × 350g jar tomato and herb pasta sauce
1 × 220g can beansprouts
1 × 415g can lentil and vegetable soup
1 small pack frozen peas

Prepacked foods
1 ready meal of your choice (max. 400 kcal)
1 pack Rosemary Conley Low Fat Belgian Chocolate Mousse
1 box Rosemary Conley Low Gi Nutrition Bars
1 prepacked low-fat sandwich (or buy fresh on day)

Store cupboard
Check if you have these and add them to your shopping list, if
necessary:

Basmati rice
Black pepper
Branston pickle

Chilli powder or chilli paste
Coffee
Cornflour
Cup-a-Soups
Garlic paste/purée
Honey
Low-calorie, low-fat salad dressing
Low-fat gravy granules or gravy powder (e.g. Bisto)
Marmite
Spaghetti
Sugar or low-calorie sugar substitute
Teabags
Vegetable stock cubes

Solo Slim Kick-start Diet menu planner

DAY 1

Breakfast
40g (1½oz) porridge oats made into porridge using water and served with 1 tsp honey and milk from allowance

Mid-morning Power Snack
1 satsuma

Lunch
1 large sweet potato baked in its jacket and topped with 50g (2oz) low-fat cottage cheese mixed with 50g (2oz) 0% fat Greek-style yogurt (e.g. Total 0%), chopped chives, ½ each chopped green, red and yellow pepper, freshly ground black pepper and unlimited green salad with oil-free dressing

Mid-afternoon Power Snack
1 kiwi fruit

Dinner
Low-fat spaghetti carbonara made with 115g (4oz) boiled spaghetti, drained and tossed with 75g (3oz) cooked chopped lean bacon, ground black pepper, chopped parsley, 3 tbsps half-fat creme fraîche and 1 tbsp grated Parmesan cheese.

DAY 2

Breakfast
2 Weetabix served with milk from allowance and 2 tsps sugar

Mid-morning Power Snack
115g (4oz) grapes

Lunch
2 slices wholegrain bread spread with low-calorie salad dressing, made into open sandwiches with 25g (1oz) wafer thin ham or 50g (2oz) canned tuna, and topped with sliced cherry tomatoes, cucumber and mixed salad leaves. Season with freshly ground black pepper to taste

Mid-afternoon Power Snack
115g (4oz) strawberries

Dinner
Chop 1 × 150g (5oz) skinned and boned chicken breast and dry-fry in a non-stick wok until almost cooked. Add ½ tsp garlic purée and stir well, then add 3 sticks chopped celery, ½ chopped pepper, ½ chopped onion, 4 chopped mushrooms and plenty of freshly ground black pepper. Add ½ jar sweet and sour stir-fry sauce and heat through. Serve with 60g (2½oz) [uncooked weight] basmati rice cooked in boiling water with a stock cube

DAY 3

Breakfast
½ fresh grapefruit plus 1 boiled egg and 1 slice
wholegrain bread spread with Marmite

Mid-morning Power Snack
1 kiwi fruit

Lunch
Turkey Spaghetti (see recipe, page 197) served with a side
salad tossed in oil-free dressing

Mid-afternoon Power Snack
115g (4oz) strawberries

Dinner
1 × 115g (4oz) salmon steak, grilled, steamed or
microwaved, served with 100g (3½oz) boiled new
potatoes (with skins), 115g (4oz) frozen peas, 200g (7oz)
broccoli and low-fat sauce of your choice

DAY 4

Breakfast
1 tbsp muesli mixed with 100g (3½oz) 0% fat Greek-style yogurt (e.g. Total 0%) and 50ml (2fl oz) milk from allowance, topped with 1 small sliced banana

Mid-morning Power Snack
½ × 35g Rosemary Conley Low Gi Nutrition Bar (any flavour)

Lunch
1 × 415g can lentil and vegetable soup (max. 250 kcal) plus 1 small piece fruit

Mid-afternoon Power Snack
½ × 35g Rosemary Conley Low Gi Nutrition Bar (any flavour)

Dinner
Chicken and beansprout stir-fry: chop 1 × 150g (5oz) skinned and boned chicken breast and dry-fry in a non-stick wok with lots of freshly ground black pepper. When the chicken is almost cooked, add 1 can beansprouts, drained, and ½ jar sweet and sour stir-fry sauce and heat through. Serve with 60g (2½oz) [uncooked weight] basmati rice cooked in boiling water with a vegetable stock cube

DAY 5

Breakfast
½ grapefruit; 3 turkey rashers, grilled, served with 1 small can plum tomatoes and 1 small can mushrooms or 25g (1oz) grilled fresh mushrooms plus ½ slice toasted wholegrain bread

Mid-morning Power Snack
1 satsuma

Lunch
1 prepacked low-fat sandwich (max. 250 kcal) plus 1 piece fruit

Mid-afternoon Power Snack
1 kiwi fruit

Dinner
1 low-fat ready meal (max. 400 kcal)

DAY 6

Breakfast
40g (1½oz) muesli served with milk from allowance and 1 tsp sugar

Mid-morning Power Snack
115g (4oz) grapes

Lunch
1 slice toasted wholegrain bread topped with 1 small can baked beans; 1 small banana

Mid-afternoon Power Snack
1 satsuma

Dinner
1 large sweet potato baked in its skin, then topped with ½ small can tuna mixed with low-fat salad dressing and 2 tbsps sweetcorn kernels, and served with a large salad tossed in oil-free dressing or 350g (12oz) boiled or steamed vegetables

DAY 7

Breakfast
1 poached egg served on 1 slice toasted wholegrain bread;
1 satsuma

Mid-morning Power Snack
1 kiwi fruit

Lunch
1 small banana, 1 × 110g Rosemary Conley Belgian
Chocolate Mousse plus 115g (4oz) strawberries

Mid-afternoon Power Snack
1 low-fat Cup-a-Soup

Dinner
1 × 150g (5oz) skinned chicken breast or 150g (6oz)
white fish, sprinkled with freshly ground black pepper, and
grilled, steamed or baked in foil. Serve with carrots,
broccoli, 115g (4oz) boiled new potatoes (with skins) and
low-fat gravy or sauce of your choice

Week 3 onwards

Remember, when you've completed the two-week Kick-start Diet, move on to Part 2 of the diet. Check the BMR charts at the back of this book to find out your personal calorie allowance. If the calories allow, add 100 calories each for your alcoholic drink, dessert and treat each day. If your BMR is greater than 1500, you can also increase your portion sizes (see page 115 for ideas on how to do this).

13 Recipes

Ⓥ means suitable for vegetarians

❄ means suitable for home freezing

Soups

Chilli bean soup Ⓥ ❄

SERVES 4
1 SERVING 163 KCAL/2.7G FAT
PREPARATION TIME 10 MINUTES
COOKING TIME 25 MINUTES

1 medium red onion, finely chopped
1 small red chilli, sliced
1 × 225g can chickpeas, drained and rinsed
1 × 225g can red kidney beans, drained and rinsed
1 large can chopped tomatoes
600ml (1 pint) vegetable stock
1 tbsp tomato purée
2 tsps chopped fresh oregano
salt and freshly ground black pepper

1 Preheat a non-stick wok or frying pan. Add the onion and
   chilli and dry-fry for 4–5 minutes.
2 Transfer to a saucepan and add the remaining ingredients.
   Simmer gently for 20 minutes. Season to taste with salt and
   pepper before serving.

Roast pepper gazpacho ⓥ

SERVES 4
1 SERVING 40 KCAL/0.4G FAT
PREPARATION TIME 20 MINUTES
COOKING TIME 10 MINUTES

2 red peppers, seeded
1 cucumber, peeled
7 celery sticks
1 garlic clove, crushed
600ml (1 pint) tomato juice
2 tsps vegetable stock powder
1 tbsp red wine vinegar
2–3 drops Tabasco sauce
salt and freshly ground black pepper
good bunch of fresh mint leaves to garnish

1 Place the red peppers on a non-stick baking tray, skin-side
   up, and cook under a hot grill until the skin blisters and
   blackens. Place in a plastic bag, seal, and allow to cool. Peel
   away the skin and discard.
2 Place the pepper flesh in a food processor. Add the
   cucumber, 3 celery sticks (reserve 4 for the garnish), garlic,
   tomato juice and stock powder. Blend until smooth, then
   pass through a metal sieve. Add the vinegar and Tabasco.
   Adjust the consistency with a little cold water and season
   with salt and black pepper. Refrigerate until ready to serve.
3 Serve in glass dishes and garnish each with mint leaves and a
   stick of celery.

Prawn noodle soup

SERVES 2
1 SERVING 92 KCAL/2.1G FAT
PREPARATION TIME 20 MINUTES
COOKING TIME 20 MINUTES

*This spicy wholesome soup makes a great winter warmer. If you
have to buy fresh spices such as lemongrass or ginger in large
quantities, prepare them then place in food bags and freeze for
a later time.*

2 spring onions, finely sliced
¼ tsp coriander seeds
½ clove smoked garlic, crushed
1 tsp finely chopped lemongrass
small piece of fresh ginger, peeled and finely chopped
pinch of dried chilli flakes
pinch of ground turmeric
300ml (½ pint) vegetable stock
25g (1oz) [uncooked weight] egg noodles
6 large uncooked prawns, peeled
25g (1oz) beansprouts
mint leaves to garnish

1 Preheat a large non-stick pan, add the spring onions and
   dry-fry until soft.
2 Crush the coriander seeds on a chopping board with the
   broad side of a chopping knife and add to the pan. Add the
   garlic and cook for 2 minutes.
3 Add the lemongrass, ginger, chilli flakes and turmeric and stir
   well to combine the spices.

4 Add the vegetable stock and bring to the boil. Reduce the heat to a gentle simmer and add the noodles. Cook for 5–6 minutes until the noodles become soft, then add the prawns as these will take only a minute to cook.
5 Remove from the heat and stir in the beansprouts. Garnish with mint leaves before serving.

Thai chicken soup

SERVES 4
1 SERVING 199 KCAL/10G FAT
PREPARATION TIME 15 MINUTES
COOKING TIME 20 MINUTES

2 chicken breasts, skinned and boned
2 small shallots, finely sliced
1 tsp coriander seeds
2 smoked garlic cloves, crushed
2 tsps finely chopped lemongrass
small piece fresh ginger, peeled and finely chopped
1 Thai red chilli, sliced
300ml (½ pint) reduced-fat coconut milk
900ml (1½ pints) vegetable stock
4 ripe tomatoes, cut into quarters
1 tbsp chopped fresh coriander leaves

1 Cut the chicken into thin strips.
2 Preheat a large non-stick pan or wok, add the chicken and shallots and dry-fry for 5–6 minutes, until firm.

3 Crush the coriander seeds on a chopping board with the broad side of a chopping knife and add to the pan along with the garlic. Cook for 2–3 minutes, and then add the lemongrass, ginger, and chilli, stirring well to combine the spices.
4 Add the coconut milk and the stock and bring to the boil. Reduce the heat and simmer gently for 5 minutes.
5 Just before serving, remove from the heat and stir in the tomato quarters and coriander leaves.

Carrot and parsnip soup Ⓥ ❄

SERVES 4
1 SERVING 160 KCAL/2.7G FAT
PREPARATION TIME 20 MINUTES
COOKING TIME 30 MINUTES

This double soup can be made a day in advance. The basic soup is suitable for freezing, although the parsley cream is not.

450g (1lb) fresh young carrots
450g (1lb) young parsnips
2 celery sticks, sliced
2 medium onions, chopped
2 garlic cloves, crushed
2 tsps chopped fresh lemon or thyme
1.2 litres (2 pints) vegetable stock
2 bay leaves
salt and freshly ground black pepper

for the parsley cream
2 tbsps virtually fat free fromage frais
1 tbsp chopped fresh parsley

1 Wash the carrots and parsnips well. Remove the tops, peel both vegetables and then slice them. Place in two separate saucepans. Divide the celery, onion, garlic and lemon or thyme between the two pans. Add the vegetable stock and the bay leaves and simmer gently until the vegetables are soft.
2 Remove the bay leaves and liquidise each soup separately until smooth, rinsing out the liquidiser between soups. Return each soup to its original pan to reheat. Adjust the consistency with a little extra stock if required and season with salt and black pepper.
3 Mix together the fromage frais and parsley, and season well with salt and black pepper, adding a little cold water to thin it down.
4 To serve, pour the soups into two identically sized jugs and then pour simultaneously into each dish to keep the colours separate. Swirl the parsley cream on top.

Seafood chowder

SERVES 4
1 SERVING 225 KCAL/1.2G FAT
PREPARATION TIME 40 MINUTES
COOKING TIME 35 MINUTES

2 onions, finely chopped
2 garlic cloves, crushed
600ml (1 pint) vegetable stock
2 tbsps plain flour
1 × 400g can chopped tomatoes
1 small red chilli, seeded and finely chopped
300ml (½ pint) tomato passata
450g (1lb) ready-to-eat seafood selection
1 tbsp chopped fresh parsley
1 tbsp chopped fresh chives
2 tbsps virtually fat free fromage frais
salt and freshly ground black pepper

1 Preheat a large non-stick saucepan, add the onion and dry-fry until soft.
2 Add the garlic and 3 tbsps of stock. Sprinkle the flour over and beat well with a wooden spoon. Cook for 1 minute in order to 'cook out' the flour, then gradually stir in the remaining stock.
3 Add the chopped tomatoes, chilli and passata and simmer gently for 10–15 minutes.
4 Stir in the seafood and herbs and remove the pan from the heat. Add the fromage frais and season to taste with salt and black pepper.

Meat

Creamy Madeira beef

SERVES 4
1 SERVING 307 KCAL/10G FAT
PREPARATION TIME 20 MINUTES
COOKING TIME 40 MINUTES

4 lean braising steaks
1 medium red onion, finely chopped
1 × 2.5cm (1in) piece fresh ginger, peeled and finely chopped
1 beef stock cube dissolved in 300ml (½ pint) water
1 tbsp plain flour
225g (8oz) chestnut mushrooms, sliced
1 wine glass Madeira wine
2 tbsps chopped fresh mixed herbs
salt and freshly ground black pepper

1 Preheat a non-stick frying pan. Season the steaks on both
   sides with salt and black pepper and place in the pan. Dry-
   fry on both sides for 5–6 minutes until lightly browned.
   Remove from the pan and place on a plate.
2 Add the onion to the pan and cook gently until lightly
   coloured. Add the ginger and 2 tbsps of stock. Sprinkle over
   the flour and 'cook out' for 1 minute. Gradually stir in the
   remaining stock. Add the mushrooms and wine.
3 Return the beef to the pan and add the herbs. Simmer gently
   for 35–40 minutes until the sauce has reduced and the beef
   is tender.

Griddled beef with Provençal vegetables

SERVES 4
1 SERVING 249 KCAL/6.6G FAT
PREPARATION TIME 20 MINUTES
COOKING TIME 20 MINUTES

4 lean pieces steak, rump or sirloin
2 red onions, cut into wedges
2 garlic cloves, crushed
1 red pepper, seeded and diced
2 courgettes, diced
1 aubergine, diced
1 × 400g can chopped tomatoes
1 tbsp chopped fresh herbs (thyme, oregano, basil)
salt and freshly ground black pepper

1 Preheat the oven to 200C, 400F, Gas Mark 6.
2 Trim any fat from the meat and discard. Season the steaks
   with salt and black pepper.
3 Preheat a non-stick frying pan or wok. Add the beef to the
   hot pan and seal very quickly on both sides. Transfer to a
   baking tray and place in the oven for 8–10 minutes to
   continue cooking.
4 Return the pan to the heat, add the onions and garlic and
   dry-fry for 2–3 minutes until they start to colour. Add the red
   pepper, courgettes and aubergine, season with salt and
   pepper and cook quickly, moving the vegetables around the
   pan with a wooden spoon. Add the tomatoes and herbs to
   the pan, stir well and simmer gently.

5 Remove the beef from the oven and allow to rest for 5 minutes.
6 Spoon the vegetables into a warm serving dish. Carve the beef into slices and arrange on top.

Beef and potato goulash ❄

SERVES 4
1 SERVING 291 KCAL/5.9G FAT
PREPARATION TIME 15 MINUTES
COOKING TIME 1 HOUR 30 MINUTES

2 medium onions, diced
2 garlic cloves, crushed
450g (1lb) lean beef steak, diced
1 tbsp plain flour
2 tsps paprika
1.2 litres (2 pints) meat stock
2 tbsps tomato purée
2 bay leaves
450g (1lb) small charlotte potatoes
2 celery sticks, chopped
1 red pepper, seeded and diced
salt and freshly ground black pepper
2 tbsps chopped fresh parsley
yogurt to serve

1 Preheat a non-stick frying pan or wok, add the onions and garlic and dry-fry for 2–3 minutes until soft.
2 Add the beef, season with salt and freshly ground black pepper, and continue to cook over a high heat until well sealed.

3 Sprinkle the flour and paprika over and 'cook out' for 1 minute.
4 Gradually stir in the stock. Add the tomato purée and bay leaves, cover, and simmer gently for 1 hour or until the meat is tender.
5 Add the potatoes, celery and red pepper and cook for a further 25 minutes.
6 Sprinkle with the chopped fresh parsley and drizzle the yogurt on top before serving.

Roast beef with Yorkshire pudding and dry-roast sweet potatoes

SERVES 6
1 SERVING BEEF: 218 KCAL/8.3G FAT; DRY-ROAST SWEET POTATOES: 67 KCAL/0.7G FAT; YORKSHIRE PUDDING: 79 KCAL/1.3G FAT
PREPARATION TIME 30 MINUTES
COOKING TIME 1–1½ HOURS

1 × 1kg (2lb) joint lean beef (topside)
1 onion, finely diced
1 carrot, diced
1 celery stick, diced
2 tsps mixed dried herbs
600ml (1 pint) beef stock
1 tbsp cornflour
1–2 drops gravy browning

for the dry-roast sweet potatoes
450g (1lb) sweet potatoes, cut in half
1 tbsp soy sauce diluted in 2 tbsps water (optional)

for the Yorkshire pudding batter
115g (4oz) plain flour
1 egg
pinch of salt
150ml (¼ pint) skimmed milk

1 Preheat the oven to 180C, 350F, Gas Mark 4.
2 Prepare the beef by removing as much visible fat as possible.
3 Place the onion, carrot, celery and herbs in the bottom of a roasting tin or ovenproof dish, sit the beef on top and pour 300ml (½ pint) water around. Place in the oven. Allow 15 minutes per 450g (1lb) plus 15 minutes over for rare beef, 20 minutes per 450g (1lb) plus 20 minutes over for medium rare, and 25 minutes per 450g (1lb) plus 30 minutes over if you like your beef well done.
4 Cook the sweet potatoes in boiling water. Drain and place in a non-stick roasting tin. Place in the top of the oven for 35–40 minutes until golden brown. You can baste them with the diluted soy sauce if they appear to dry out.
5 Forty minutes before the beef is ready, make the batter by blending the flour with the egg and a little milk to a smooth paste. Add the salt and whisk in the remaining milk until smooth. Preheat a six-hole, non-stick Yorkshire pudding tin for 2 minutes in the oven. Remove and half-fill each mould with batter. Increase the oven temperature to 200C, 400F, Gas Mark 6, place the pudding batter in the oven and cook for 35–40 minutes.
6 When the beef is cooked, remove it from the roasting tin and wrap in foil to keep warm. Allow it to rest for 5–10 minutes. Meanwhile, add the beef stock to the pan juices, slake the cornflour with a little water and add to the pan. Stir well as

the gravy thickens and add 1–2 drops of gravy browning as required.

7 To serve, carve the beef thinly. Serve with the Yorkshire puddings, dry-roast sweet potatoes, gravy and seasonal vegetables.

Beef masala ❄

SERVES 4
1 SERVING 349 KCAL/12G FAT
PREPARATION TIME 10 MINUTES
COOKING TIME 1½ HOURS

For a creamy curry, add 2 tbsps of virtually fat free fromage frais just before serving.

2 red onions, diced
2 garlic cloves, crushed
1kg (2lb) lean beef steak, diced
1 tsp cumin seeds
1 tsp coriander seeds
1 tsp ground cardamom
4 whole cloves
1 × 2.5cm (1in) piece of ginger, peeled and chopped
2 small red chillies
2 × 400g cans chopped tomatoes
2 beef stock cubes
2 tbsps tomato purée
1 cinnamon stick
salt and freshly ground black pepper
chopped fresh parsley or mint to garnish

1 Preheat a non-stick wok or deep frying pan. Add the onions and garlic and dry-fry for 2–3 minutes until soft. Add the beef and season with salt and black pepper. Continue to cook over a high heat until well sealed. Sprinkle the spices over the meat and 'cook out' for 1 minute.

2 Stir in the remaining ingredients, cover and simmer gently for 1 hour or until the meat is tender, adding a little water if required.

3 Just before serving sprinkle with chopped fresh parsley or mint.

Fillet steak with redcurrant and thyme glaze

SERVES 4
1 SERVING 215 KCAL/6G FAT
PREPARATION TIME 10 MINUTES
COOKING TIME 20 MINUTES

4 × 150g (4 × 5oz) rump steaks
2 tbsps redcurrant jelly
1 tsp chopped fresh thyme
150ml (¼ pint) vegetable stock
salt and freshly ground black pepper

1 Preheat a non-stick frying pan. Season the steaks on both sides with salt and black pepper. Add to the pan and seal for 2–3 minutes on each side. Continue cooking for a further 5 minutes, turning the steaks regularly. Remove from the pan and keep warm.

2 Add the redcurrant jelly, thyme and stock to the pan and mix
   well. Simmer gently to allow the sauce to thicken then return
   the steaks to the pan. Serve hot.

Pastrami hotpot

SERVES 4
1 SERVING 259 KCAL/5G FAT
PREPARATION TIME 10 MINUTES
COOKING TIME 50 MINUTES

8 slices pastrami
8 long shallots, peeled
300ml (½ pint) red wine
300ml (½ pint) water
pinch of fresh thyme
2 tbsps gravy granules
4 large potatoes, peeled and sliced very thin
olive oil spray (e.g. Fry Light)

1 Preheat the oven to180C, 350F, Gas Mark 4.
2 Wrap a slice of pastrami around each shallot and place in the
   bottom of an ovenproof dish.
3 Pour the wine and water into a saucepan. Add the thyme and
   bring to the boil. Stir in the gravy granules and allow to
   thicken. Pour the gravy over the meat, cover with the sliced
   potatoes and lightly spray with olive oil spray.
4 Place in the oven for 40 minutes until the potatoes are
   cooked through.

Quick sausage casserole

SERVES 4
1 SERVING 234 KCAL/7.5G FAT
PREPARATION TIME 15 MINUTES
COOKING TIME 25 MINUTES

For extra flavour, you can add 1 tsp red chilli paste along with the canned tomatoes.

1 × 400g pack low-fat sausages
1 onion, chopped
1 garlic clove, crushed
½ red and ½ green pepper, seeded and chopped
½ medium courgette, chopped
1 × 415g can baked beans
1 × 400g can chopped tomatoes
1 tsp red chilli paste (optional)
2 tsps Worcester sauce
1 tsp tomato purée
1 tsp mixed herbs
freshly ground black pepper

1 Grill the sausages until brown and cooked through.
2 Meanwhile, preheat a non-stick frying pan. Add the onion and garlic and dry-fry for 1 minute. Add the peppers and courgette, cover and continue cooking for a further 2 minutes.
3 When the vegetables are soft, add the baked beans, chopped tomatoes, chilli paste (if using), Worcester sauce, tomato purée and herbs and mix well. Simmer over a low heat for 10 minutes.

4 When cooked, cut the sausages into chunks and add to the vegetable and sauce mixture. Simmer for a further 5 minutes, and add ground black pepper to taste.

Sweet chilli pork

SERVES 4
1 SERVING 241 KCAL/4.9G FAT
PREPARATION TIME 10 MINUTES
COOKING TIME 25 MINUTES

4 lean pork steaks
2 garlic cloves, finely chopped
50ml (2fl oz) dry sherry
2 tsps runny honey
1 × 400g can chopped tomatoes
1 red chilli, finely sliced
1 tsp ground coriander
salt and freshly ground black pepper
fresh coriander to serve

1 Trim away any fat from the pork and discard. Season the pork well with salt and black pepper and set aside.
2 Preheat a non-stick frying pan until hot. Carefully add the pork and turn quickly to seal all sides.
3 Add the garlic and allow to soften.
4 Add the sherry and the remaining ingredients. Simmer gently for 20 minutes until the pork is cooked through.
5 Arrange the pork on a serving plate and pour the sauce over. Sprinkle with fresh coriander.

Pork and pineapple kebabs

SERVES 4
1 SERVING 309 KCAL/6G FAT
PREPARATION TIME 20 MINUTES
COOKING TIME 25 MINUTES

4 lean pork steaks
1 large pineapple
2 garlic cloves, finely chopped
1 small chilli, sliced
2 tbsps maple syrup
salt and freshly ground black pepper

1 Trim any fat off the pork steaks and discard. Cut the steaks into bite-sized pieces.
2 Prepare the pineapple by slicing off the top and bottom with a sharp knife. Cut away the sides to leave a barrel-shaped fruit. Cut into slices, then into small wedges.
3 Take eight wooden kebab skewers and thread alternate pieces of pork and pineapple on to each. Place in a shallow dish.
4 Mix together the garlic, chilli and maple syrup and pour over the kebabs. Season with salt and black pepper.
5 Place under a hot grill for 20–25 minutes until fully cooked.

Spicy meatballs with spaghetti

SERVES 4
1 SERVING 469 KCAL/12G FAT
PREPARATION TIME 10 MINUTES
COOKING TIME 30 MINUTES

450g (1lb) lean minced pork
225g (8oz) low-fat sausage meat
2 garlic cloves, crushed
2 tsps vegetable stock powder
1 tsp paprika
1 small red chilli, finely chopped
1 tsp Italian herb seasoning
1 tbsp finely chopped fresh parsley
225g (8oz) [uncooked weight] spaghetti
freshly grated Parmesan cheese to garnish

for the sauce
1 × 690g bottle tomato passata
6 basil leaves

1 Place both meats in a large mixing bowl with the garlic, stock powder, paprika, chilli, Italian herb seasoning and parsley and mix well. Form the mixture into 24 balls.
2 Preheat a non-stick frying pan. Add the meatballs and cook over a moderate heat for 10 minutes to brown the outsides. Drain away any fat, then add the passata and allow to simmer for 10 minutes.
3 Meanwhile cook the spaghetti in a large pan of boiling water. Drain well and pour into a large serving dish.

4 Finely shred the basil, add to the sauce and spoon over the spaghetti.
5 Garnish with a little Parmesan before serving.

Lemon and honey glazed pork steaks

SERVES 4
1 SERVING 241 KCAL/4.8G FAT
PREPARATION TIME 10 MINUTES
COOKING TIME 30 MINUTES

4 lean pork steaks
zest and juice of 2 lemons
2 tbsps runny honey
2 garlic cloves, crushed
2 tsps chopped fresh rosemary
salt and freshly ground black pepper

1 Remove all the fat from the pork steaks with a sharp knife and discard. Place the steaks in a shallow container. Season on both sides with salt and black pepper.
2 Combine the remaining ingredients in a small bowl and mix well. Pour over the pork and turn the steaks over to coat both sides.
3 Cook under a hot grill for 8–10 minutes on each side, basting with more glaze if required. Serve hot.

Italian shepherd's pie ❄

SERVES 4
1 SERVING 400 KCAL/9G FAT
PREPARATION TIME 60 MINUTES
COOKING TIME 30 MINUTES

Try this traditional family dish with a Mediterranean-style twist.
Delicious!

450g (1lb) extra lean minced lamb
1 medium red onion, finely chopped
2 garlic cloves, crushed
225g (8oz) chestnut mushrooms, finely sliced
1 tbsp chopped fresh oregano
2 tsps vegetable bouillon stock powder
2 × 400g cans chopped tomatoes
1kg (2lb) potatoes
3 leeks, trimmed and finely chopped
8 sun-dried tomatoes, finely chopped
olive oil spray (e.g. Fry Light)
salt and freshly ground black pepper

1 Preheat the oven to 200C, 400F, Gas Mark 6. Preheat a non-
   stick saucepan.
2 Add the lamb, onion and garlic to the hot pan and brown
   quickly over a high heat. Add the mushrooms, oregano and
   stock powder, stirring well. Pour in the tomatoes and simmer
   gently for 20 minutes to allow the meat to cook and the
   sauce to reduce.

3 Meanwhile, cook the potatoes in a saucepan of salted boiling water. Drain and mash well until smooth. Add the leeks and sun-dried tomatoes and mix well. Season with salt and black pepper.
4 Using a slotted spoon, place the meat mixture in the bottom of an ovenproof dish. Cover with the potatoes, smooth over with a fork and spray lightly with olive oil spray.
5 Bake in the oven for 30–40 minutes until golden.

Lamb chasseur

SERVES 4
1 SERVING 328 KCAL/11G FAT
PREPARATION TIME 15 MINUTES
COOKING TIME 40 MINUTES

Allow the meat to stand for 10 minutes after cooking. This allows the joint to relax and makes it easier to carve.

450g (1lb) leg of lamb, fat removed
2 medium red onions, sliced
2 garlic cloves, crushed
150ml (¼ pint) vegetable stock
1 tbsp plain flour
150ml (¼ pint) red wine
1 × 400g can chopped tomatoes
1 tbsp chopped fresh tarragon
115g (4oz) button mushrooms
salt and freshly ground black pepper

1 Preheat the oven to 180C, 350F, Gas Mark 4.
2 Preheat a non-stick frying pan until very hot. Add the lamb and quickly brown on all sides, then transfer the meat to an earthenware dish.
3 Add the onions and garlic to the frying pan and cook until lightly coloured. Add 2–3 tbsps of stock and sprinkle the flour over. Cook briefly then gradually mix in the remaining stock, wine and chopped tomatoes. Bring to the boil and stir in the tarragon and mushrooms. Season with salt and black pepper. Pour the sauce over the lamb and cover with a lid.
4 Place in the oven and bake for 40 minutes until tender.
5 Before serving, scoop any fat from the top of the dish with a small ladle, then remove the meat from the sauce and place on a serving plate. Adjust the consistency of the sauce by reducing in a saucepan over a high heat. Serve the lamb with the sauce.

Chicken and poultry

Spicy lemon chicken

SERVES 2
1 SERVING 292 KCAL/6G FAT
PREPARATION TIME 10 MINUTES
MARINATING TIME 1 HOUR
COOKING TIME 15 MINUTES

450g (1lb) chicken breasts, skinned and boned
zest and juice of 1 lemon
2 tbsps light soy sauce
1 tsp ground coriander
150ml (¼ pint) tomato passata
1 small red chilli, finely sliced
1 tsp finely chopped lemongrass
2 garlic cloves, crushed
salt and freshly ground black pepper
1 tbsp chopped fresh coriander

1 Cut the chicken into cubes and place in a shallow dish.
   Season with salt and pepper. Combine the remaining
   ingredients, except the fresh coriander, and pour over the
   chicken. Marinate for at least 1 hour, mixing occasionally.
2 Strain away the marinade from the chicken and reserve.
   Preheat a non-stick wok or frying pan and dry-fry the
   chicken quickly over a high heat for 5–6 minutes, turning it
   to seal all sides.
3 Add the reserved marinade and continue to cook for a
   further 10 minutes, to allow the sauce to simmer gently and
   thicken. Stir in the fresh coriander and serve.

Tomato, chicken and ginger stir-fry ❄

SERVES 4
1 SERVING 307 KCAL/3.3G FAT
PREPARATION TIME 15 MINUTES
COOKING TIME 20 MINUTES
MARINATING TIME 1 HOUR

4 chicken breasts, skinned and boned
2 tbsps dry sherry
zest and juice of 1 orange
2 tbsps runny honey
2 tbsps fruit chutney
2 garlic cloves, crushed
1 tsp finely chopped ginger
1 tbsp tomato purée
1 red pepper, seeded and sliced
1 yellow pepper, seeded and sliced
salt and freshly ground black pepper

1 Cut the chicken into long, thin strips and place in a shallow
   dish. Season with salt and black pepper.
2 Combine the sherry, orange zest and juice, honey and
   chutney, mix well and add the garlic, ginger and tomato
   purée. Pour the mixture over the chicken, cover and
   refrigerate for 1 hour to marinate.
3 Preheat a non-stick wok or large frying pan. Lift the chicken
   pieces from the marinade, add to the pan and cook quickly
   over a high heat for 5–6 minutes. Add the peppers and
   continue cooking for a further 5–6 minutes until the chicken
   is cooked through. Add any remaining marinade and allow to
   heat through.

Garlicky chicken Kiev ❄

SERVES 4
1 SERVING 351 KCAL/11G FAT
PREPARATION TIME 10 MINUTES
COOKING TIME 30 MINUTES

4 chicken breasts, skinned
50g (2oz) low-fat spread
2 garlic cloves, crushed
1 tbsp finely chopped fresh chives
salt and freshly ground black pepper
2 tbsps flour
1 egg, beaten
4 tbsps cornmeal

1 Preheat the oven to 200C, 400F, Gas Mark 6.
2 Place the chicken breasts on a chopping board and slice
   through the centre of each to make a pocket.
3 Mix the low-fat spread with the garlic and chives and season
   with salt and black pepper. Distribute the garlic spread
   between the chicken breasts, spooning into the pocket of
   each chicken breast.
4 Roll the chicken breasts in the flour, then the beaten egg
   and finally the cornmeal. Place on a non-stick baking tray.
5 Bake in the oven for 25–30 minutes until cooked through.
   Serve hot.

Cheesy bacon chicken

SERVES 4
1 SERVING 284 KCAL/9G FAT
PREPARATION TIME 10 MINUTES
COOKING TIME 30 MINUTES

4 chicken breasts, skinned
2 × 150g (2 × 5oz) reduced-fat mozzarella, sliced
8 basil leaves
4 slices Parma ham

1 Preheat the oven to 200C, 400F, Gas Mark 6.
2 Place the chicken breasts on a chopping board and slice
   through the centre of each to make a pocket. Distribute the
   cheese and the basil leaves between the pockets. Wrap the
   Parma ham around the outside of each breast and place on a
   non-stick baking tray.
3 Bake in the oven for 25–30 minutes until cooked through.
   Serve hot.

Green Thai chicken curry

SERVES 4
1 SERVING 244 KCAL/4G FAT
PREPARATION TIME 25 MINUTES
COOKING TIME 30 MINUTES

2 red onions
3 garlic cloves, chopped
4 chicken breasts, skinned and boned
1 tbsp ground coriander
½ tsp ground turmeric
¼ tsp fenugreek seeds or ground fenugreek
1 small fresh red chilli, chopped
seeds from 4 cardamom pods
4 kaffir lime leaves (optional)
300ml (½ pint) chicken stock
300ml (½ pint) reduced-fat coconut milk
2 tbsps chopped fresh basil
115g (4oz) shredded fresh spinach
salt and freshly ground black pepper

1 Preheat a non-stick wok or frying pan. Dry-fry the onions and garlic until soft and lightly coloured.
2 Cut the chicken into dice, add to the pan and seal the outside of the meat. Season with salt and black pepper. Add the spices and kaffir lime leaves (if using) and continue cooking for 2 minutes before adding the stock, coconut milk and basil.
3 Reduce the heat and allow to simmer gently as the sauce thickens. Just before serving stir in the spinach.

Chicken with tangerine and cinnamon

SERVES 4
1 SERVING 263 KCAL/4.4G FAT
PREPARATION TIME 40 MINUTES
COOKING TIME 35 MINUTES

4 chicken breasts, skinned
4 tangerines
300ml (½ pint) fresh apple juice
2 garlic cloves, crushed
2 cinnamon sticks
1 tbsp fresh thyme
1 tbsp plum sauce
2 tsps sweet grain mustard
150ml (¼ pint) chicken stock
2 tbsps tomato purée
sea salt and freshly ground black pepper

1 Preheat the oven to 170C, 325F, Gas Mark 3. Preheat a non-stick frying pan.
2 Season the chicken breasts on both sides with salt and black pepper. Add to the pan and brown on both sides. Transfer to an ovenproof dish.
3 Cut the tangerines in half and squeeze the juice over the chicken.
4 Mix together the remaining ingredients and pour over the chicken. Cover with a lid or foil and bake in the oven for 30 minutes until the chicken is fully cooked.

Chicken with lime and ginger

SERVES 4
1 SERVING 266 KCAL/7G FAT
PREPARATION TIME 10 MINUTES
COOKING TIME 20 MINUTES

4 chicken breasts, skinned and boned
4 small leeks, trimmed and finely chopped
2 garlic cloves, crushed
1 × 2.5cm (1in) piece fresh ginger, finely chopped
1 tsp ground cumin
1 tsp lemongrass paste
150ml (¼ pint) chicken stock
zest and juice of 1 lime
225g (8oz) half-fat crème fraîche
salt and freshly ground black pepper
1 tbsp chopped fresh coriander

1 Cut the chicken into thin strips and season with salt and black pepper.
2 Preheat a non-stick frying pan. Add the chicken and cook until lightly browned. Add the leeks, garlic, ginger, cumin and lemongrass paste and continue to cook over a low heat for 2 minutes.
3 Add the chicken stock and the lime zest and juice and bring to a gentle simmer.
4 Fold in the crème fraîche and bring back to the boil.
5 Just before serving sprinkle with chopped fresh coriander.

Caribbean chicken skewers with mango salsa

SERVES 4
1 SERVING 217 KCAL/5.2G FAT
PREPARATION TIME 15 MINUTES
MARINATING TIME 2 HOURS
COOKING TIME 10–15 MINUTES

1 orange
2 tbsps rum
2 tsps jerk seasoning
4 chicken breasts, skinned and boned
1 red and 1 yellow pepper, seeded
sunflower oil spray (e.g. Fry Light)

for the salsa
1 medium mango
2 tomatoes, chopped
4 spring onions, chopped

1   Grate the zest from the orange and put aside for the salsa. Squeeze the juice and pour into a bowl. Add the rum and jerk seasoning and mix together.
2   Cut the chicken into bite-sized pieces and add to the marinade. Cover and refrigerate for at least 2 hours.
3   Meanwhile, cut the peppers into 2.5cm (1in) pieces.
4   To make the salsa, peel the mango and cut into small dice. Put into a bowl with the tomatoes, spring onions and reserved orange zest. Season and stir together.
5   Thread the chicken and pepper pieces on to eight skewers and place on a grill pan. Spray each with a little sunflower oil

spray, and place under the grill for 5–7 minutes. Turn the skewers over and spray again. Continue to cook for about 5 minutes, until the chicken is tender. Serve with the mango salsa.

Chinese-style chicken

SERVES 4
1 SERVING 217 KCAL/3.6G FAT
PREPARATION TIME 10 MINUTES
COOKING TIME 20 MINUTES

4 chicken breasts, skinned and boned
8 spring onions, sliced
1 × 140g can water chestnuts, drained and sliced
1 × 5cm (2in) piece fresh ginger, peeled and sliced
1 tsp vegetable stock powder
2 tsps cornflour
600ml (1 pint) water
salt and freshly ground black pepper

1 Preheat a non-stick frying pan or wok. Cut the chicken into strips, add to the pan, and season with salt and black pepper.
2 Cook the chicken over a high heat until the flesh is lightly browned.
3 Add the spring onions, water chestnuts, ginger and stock powder.
4 Mix the cornflour with a little of the water to form a paste, then stir in the remaining water and add to the pan. Simmer gently for 5 minutes to allow the sauce to thicken. Serve hot.

Marinated barbecue chicken

SERVES 4
1 SERVING 293 KCAL/12G FAT
PREPARATION TIME 20 MINUTES
MARINATING TIME 1 HOUR
COOKING TIME 30 MINUTES

8 × 225g (8 × 8oz) chicken joints (legs and thighs)

for the marinade
2 tbsps tomato purée
2 tsps soft dark brown sugar
2 tbsps balsamic vinegar
pinch of fennel seeds
salt and freshly ground black pepper

1 Place the chicken joints on a chopping board. Pull off the
   skin, using kitchen paper and a small sharp knife, and
   discard. Place the chicken in a mixing bowl.
2 Combine the marinade ingredients in a small bowl and pour
   over the chicken. Mix well, rubbing the marinade into the
   chicken pieces. Season with salt and black pepper. Cover and
   leave to marinate in the refrigerator for an hour.
3 Cook the chicken under a hot grill for 30 minutes, turning
   regularly. Serve hot or cold.

Spicy chicken pasta

SERVES 4
1 SERVING 398 KCAL/3.3G FAT
PREPARATION TIME 10 MINUTES
COOKING TIME 20 MINUTES

225g (8oz) [uncooked weight] tagliatelle
1 vegetable stock cube
1 red onion, finely chopped
2 garlic cloves, crushed
1 red pepper, seeded and finely sliced
4 chicken breasts, skinned and boned
1 × 400g can chopped tomatoes
1 red chilli, seeded and finely chopped
8–10 basil leaves, shredded
freshly grated Parmesan
salt and freshly ground black pepper

1 Cook the pasta in boiling water with a vegetable stock cube.
2 Meanwhile, preheat a non-stick frying pan. Add the onion
   and dry-fry for 2–3 minutes until soft. Add the garlic and red
   pepper and cook for a further 2–3 minutes.
3 Cut the chicken into strips, and add to the pan. Season with
   salt and black pepper. Cook for 5 minutes until it is firm and
   changes colour. Turn the chicken during cooking so that it
   cooks on all sides.
4 Add the tomatoes and chilli and bring the sauce to a gentle
   simmer.
5 Drain the pasta and pour into a serving dish. Spoon the
   sauce over and sprinkle with shredded basil leaves and a little
   Parmesan.

Chicken and spinach lasagne

SERVES 4
1 SERVING 508 KCAL/ 8G FAT
PREPARATION TIME 25 MINUTES
COOKING TIME 25 MINUTES

4 chicken breasts, skinned and boned
1 small onion, chopped
1 small red pepper, seeded and diced
1 × 500g jar tomato pasta sauce
1 tsp chilli paste or powder
100g (3½oz) fresh spinach
6 lasagne sheets
400g low-fat white sauce (e.g. Tesco Fresh White Sauce)
50g (2oz) low-fat Cheddar cheese, grated

1 Preheat the oven to 180C, 350F, Gas Mark 4. Preheat a non-stick frying pan or wok.
2 Cut the chicken into strips and dry-fry in the non-stick pan for 5–6 minutes, until cooked. Add the onion and cook for 2 minutes. Add the red pepper and cook for a further 2 minutes. Add the pasta sauce and chilli. Simmer, uncovered, for 10 minutes, stirring occasionally. Remove from the heat.
3 Wash and roughly chop the spinach and add to the tomato and chicken mixture.
4 Place half the tomato and chicken mixture in a medium-sized lasagne dish and arrange three lasagne sheets on top. Add the remaining mixture and then the remaining lasagne sheets and top with the white sauce. Sprinkle the grated cheese on top.
5 Place in the oven and bake for 20-25 minutes.

Turkey spaghetti

SERVES 1
1 SERVING 228 KCAL/2.5G FAT
PREPARATION TIME 5 MINUTES
COOKING TIME 30 MINUTES

3 turkey rashers
50g (2oz) [uncooked weight] spaghetti
1 vegetable stock cube
1 small can chopped tomatoes
25g (1oz) button mushrooms
1 small can sweetcorn
1 tablespoon Branston pickle
2 teaspoons cornflour
salt and freshly ground black pepper

1 Grill the turkey rashers on both sides.
2 Cook the spaghetti in boiling water for 10 minutes with the vegetable stock cube.
3 While the spaghetti is cooking, place the tomatoes in a saucepan and add the mushrooms, sweetcorn and pickle. Cook on a moderate heat, then allow to simmer.
4 Snip the turkey rashers into bite-sized pieces and add to the tomato mixture.
5 Dissolve the cornflour in a little cold water and gradually add to the turkey and tomato mixture so that it thickens it as it simmers. Season to taste.
6 Drain the spaghetti, place on a serving plate and top with the turkey and tomato mixture.

Turkey and pepper burgers ❄

SERVES 4
1 SERVING 142 KCAL/2.2G FAT
PREPARATION TIME 15 MINUTES
COOKING TIME 25 MINUTES

450g (1lb) extra lean minced turkey
1 medium red onion, finely chopped
1 garlic clove, crushed
½ red pepper, finely chopped
6 basil leaves, finely chopped
2 tsps vegetable stock powder
freshly ground black pepper

1 In a large mixing bowl combine together the turkey, onion, garlic and red pepper, working the mixture with two forks to break up the meat.
2 Sprinkle the stock powder over and stir in well, making sure the mixture is fully combined.
3 Add the basil leaves and season with plenty of freshly ground black pepper. Mix well, using your hands, and bring the mixture together. Form into burger shapes, squeezing the mixture between your hands to form a tight ball and then flatten slightly. Set aside.
4 Place under a hot grill for 10 minutes each side. Pull a burger apart to check the centre is fully cooked. If in doubt, return to the grill.

Turkey Amatriciana

SERVES 1
1 SERVING 443 KCAL/2.4G FAT
PREPARATION TIME 5 MINUTES
COOKING TIME 20 MINUTES

75g (3oz) [uncooked weight] pasta shapes
½ vegetable stock cube
3 turkey rashers, chopped
½ onion, chopped
½ garlic clove, crushed
½ red pepper, chopped
1 × 400g can chopped tomatoes
½ tsp chilli powder or chilli paste
freshly ground black pepper
4 fresh basil leaves to garnish

1 Cook the pasta shapes in boiling water with the vegetable stock cube.
2 Preheat a non-stick frying pan. Add the turkey rashers, onion and garlic, and dry-fry until browned.
3 Add the red pepper and cook for a further 2 minutes. Add the chopped tomatoes, chilli and black pepper and simmer for 10 minutes.
4 When the pasta is cooked, drain and rinse and add to the sauce. Mix well, and garnish with the basil leaves before serving.

Cajun turkey with cherry tomato and roasted pepper salad

SERVES 4
1 SERVING 212 KCAL/3G FAT
PREPARATION TIME 15 MINUTES PLUS
MARINATING TIME 1 HOUR
COOKING TIME 30 MINUTES

3 thick turkey fillets (675g/1½lb total)
1 tsp dried thyme
1 tsp dried marjoram
1 tsp curry powder
1 tsp ground cumin
1 tsp ground coriander
¼ tsp chilli powder
olive oil spray (e.g. Fry Light)

for the salad
2 red peppers
250g (10oz) cherry tomatoes, quartered
1 small red onion, thinly sliced
1 red chilli, seeded and finely chopped (optional)
1 tsp red wine vinegar
salt and freshly ground black pepper

1 Thickly cut each turkey fillet to make 16 medallions in total. Mix together the herbs and spices and sprinkle over both sides of the turkey pieces. Cover and set aside for 1 hour.

2 For the salad, place the peppers under a hot grill and allow to blacken and blister all over. Transfer to a plastic bag to cool for 20 minutes, then peel off the skin and discard the seeds. Cut into dice and mix with the tomatoes, red onion, chilli (if using) and vinegar. Season with salt and black pepper.

3 Spray the turkey with a little olive oil spray on each side. Place a large heavy frying pan over a medium heat, add the turkey and cook for 4–5 minutes on each side. Serve with the tomato and pepper salad.

Fish and seafood

Spiced tomato baked cod

SERVES 4
1 SERVING 219 KCAL/2G FAT
PREPARATION TIME 15 MINUTES
COOKING TIME 15 MINUTES

1kg (2lb) thick cod fillet, skinned, boned and cut into 4 steaks
1 large red onion, finely chopped
1 garlic clove, crushed
4 ripe tomatoes, diced
1 tsp paprika
1 tsp ground turmeric
1 tsp saffron
1 tbsp chopped fresh parsley
juice of ½ lemon
salt and freshly ground black pepper

1 Preheat the oven to 200C, 400F, Gas Mark 6.
2 Season the fish well on both sides and place, skin-side down, in an ovenproof dish.
3 Preheat a non-stick pan, add the onion and dry-fry until soft. Add the garlic, tomatoes and spices and cook briskly for 4–5 minutes. Add the parsley and lemon. Season well with salt and black pepper.
4 Spoon equal amounts on to each cod steak and place, uncovered, in the hot oven for 12–15 minutes or until just cooked. When just cooked, the cod should flake easily when teased with a fork.

Thai fish cakes with dill sauce ❄

SERVES 4
1 SERVING (2 FISH CAKES) 221 KCAL/1.7G FAT
PREPARATION TIME 30 MINUTES
COOKING TIME 10 MINUTES

450g (1lb) boiling potatoes
450g (1lb) white fish, skinned and boned
4 spring onions, finely chopped
3 tsps Thai red curry paste
1 tbsp chopped fresh dill
50g (2oz) fresh breadcrumbs
olive oil spray (e.g. Fry Light)
salt and freshly ground black pepper

for the dill sauce
4 tbsps virtually fat free fromage frais
½ tsp ground turmeric
1 tbsp chopped fresh dill
2 tsps lemon juice
1 tbsp chopped fresh parsley
salt and freshly ground black pepper

1 Peel the potatoes and chop into small pieces. Place in a
   saucepan, cover with boiling water and cook until tender.
   Drain well and mash until smooth. Place in a mixing bowl.
2 Cook the fish either in a steamer above the potatoes or
   poach for 10 minutes in a little milk.
3 Allow the fish to cool, then flake the fish into the potatoes.
   Add the spring onions and red curry paste, mix well and
   season with salt and black pepper.

4 Divide the mixture into eight portions. Mix together the dill and breadcrumbs. Roll each fish cake in the breadcrumbs and dill mixture and shape with a palette knife.
5 Lightly spray a non-stick pan with olive oil spray. Add the fish cakes and dry-fry for 6 minutes on each side.
6 Place the sauce ingredients in a small bowl and mix well.
7 Serve the fish cakes hot with the dill sauce.

Baked cod with Parma ham and saffron couscous

SERVES 4
1 SERVING 361 KCAL/6.5G FAT
PREPARATION TIME 5 MINUTES
COOKING TIME 20 MINUTES

4 fresh cod fillets, skinned and boned
8 large basil leaves
8 slices Parma ham
225g (8oz) [uncooked weight] couscous
300ml (½ pint) vegetable stock
pinch of saffron
1 red pepper, seeded and finely diced
1 tbsp chopped fresh chives
salt and freshly ground black pepper

1 Preheat the oven to 200C, 400F, Gas Mark 6.
2 Place the cod fillets in an ovenproof dish. Season each fillet on both sides with salt and black pepper. Place 2 basil leaves across the top of each fillet. Wrap each piece of fish in 2 slices of Parma ham.

3 Place in the oven for 15–20 minutes until cooked through.
4 Place the couscous in a large bowl. Add the saffron and red pepper.
5 Make up the stock with boiling water and pour over the couscous. Cover with a clean tea towel and allow to stand for 1 minute. Remove the tea towel and fluff up the grains with a fork.
6 Arrange the couscous on a serving plate and place the cod fillets on top. Just before serving sprinkle with chopped fresh chives.

Mediterranean fish stew

SERVES 4
1 SERVING 255 KCAL/2.7G FAT
PREPARATION TIME 15 MINUTES
COOKING TIME 30 MINUTES

12 fresh mussels
1 onion, thinly sliced
1 garlic clove, crushed
450g (1lb) tomatoes, skinned, seeded and chopped
150ml (¼ pint) dry white wine
150ml (¼ pint) fish stock
1 tbsp chopped fresh dill
2 tbsps chopped fresh rosemary
1 tbsp tomato purée
450g (1lb) monkfish fillet, skinned and cut into large chunks
8 jumbo prawns, peeled
225g (8oz) squid, cleaned and cut into rings
salt and freshly ground black pepper

1 To clean the mussels, put in a large bowl and scrape well under cold running water (discard any that are open). Rinse until there is no trace of sand in the bowl.

2 Preheat a large non-stick saucepan, add the onion and dry-fry for 3–4 minutes. Add the garlic and tomatoes and cook for a further 3–4 minutes.

3 Add the white wine, fish stock, herbs, tomato purée and season with salt and black pepper. Bring to the boil, then lower the heat and simmer for a further 5 minutes.

4 Add the monkfish and simmer for 5 minutes. Add the prawns and squid and simmer for a further 5 minutes. Add the prepared mussels, cover the pan, and cook for 3-4 minutes until the shells open. Discard any mussels that do not open. Ladle the stew into a bowl and serve at once.

Baked salmon with tomato and lime salsa

SERVES 2
1 SERVING 380 KCAL/20G FAT
PREPARATION TIME 5 MINUTES
COOKING TIME 15 MINUTES

Sweet and sour flavours of tomato and lime add the perfect touch to this salmon dish.

2 fresh salmon fillets, skinned and boned

for the marinade
1 tbsp runny honey
zest and juice of 1 lime

1 tsp coriander seeds
1 tsp finely chopped pickled ginger
salt and freshly ground black pepper

for the salsa
4 ripe tomatoes
4 thin slices red chilli
1 tbsp finely chopped fresh chives
zest and juice of 1 lime
salt and freshly ground black pepper

1 Preheat the oven to 200C, 400F, Gas Mark 6.
2 Place the salmon fillets in an ovenproof dish and season each fillet on both sides with salt and black pepper.
3 Combine the marinade ingredients and pour over each piece of salmon. Bake in the oven for 10 minutes until just cooked.
4 Meanwhile, make the salsa by skinning the tomatoes and placing in boiling water for 10 seconds. Remove and place immediately in a bowl of iced water. Peel away the skin, cut in half and remove the seeds with a teaspoon. Chop the flesh into dice and mix with the other salsa ingredients.
5 Serve the salmon hot from the oven with the salsa on top.

Marinated griddled tuna

SERVES 4
1 SERVING 250 KCAL/8G FAT
PREPARATION TIME 45 MINUTES
COOKING TIME 10 MINUTES

4 thick tuna steaks
olive oil spray (e.g. Fry Light)
salt and freshly ground black pepper

for the marinade
4 tbsps light soy sauce
zest and juice of 2 limes
1 small red chilli, seeded and finely chopped
1 × 2.5cm (1in) piece fresh ginger, peeled and finely chopped

1 Place the tuna steaks in a shallow dish and season with black pepper.
2 Combine all the marinade ingredients in a small bowl and pour over the tuna. Leave to marinate for 30 minutes.
3 Preheat a non-stick griddle pan and lightly spray with a little olive oil spray.
4 When the pan is very hot carefully add the tuna steaks and cook quickly for 2–3 minutes on each side. Don't overcook them or the texture will become tough and dry. Serve hot.

Tuna and sweetcorn pasta

SERVES 3
1 SERVING 408 KCAL/5G FAT
PREPARATION TIME 10 MINUTES
COOKING TIME 30 MINUTES

150g (5oz) [uncooked weight] pasta shells
1 vegetable stock cube
1 medium onion, chopped
50g (2oz) mushrooms, chopped
1 × 185g can tuna in brine, drained
1 × 142g can sweetcorn, drained
1 can Campbell's Condensed 99% fat free mushroom soup
1 tbsp chopped fresh parsley
1 tsp chopped fresh dill
25g (1oz) grated low-fat Cheddar cheese
freshly ground black pepper

1 Cook the pasta in boiling water with the vegetable stock cube.
2 Preheat a non-stick pan. Add the onion and dry-fry until soft. Add the mushrooms, tuna, sweetcorn and mushroom soup and heat through, leaving to simmer gently for 5 minutes. If the sauce is too thick, add a little skimmed milk. Add the fresh herbs towards the end of cooking and season with black pepper.
3 When the pasta is cooked, drain and rinse well in boiling water. Mix into the sauce. Place in a shallow, ovenproof dish and top with the grated cheese.
4 Place under a hot grill until the cheese has melted. Serve immediately.

Fresh salmon pasta salad

SERVES 6
1 SERVING 280 KCAL/8.9G FAT
PREPARATION TIME 10 MINUTES
COOKING TIME 25 MINUTES

If fresh salmon is unavailable, canned salmon is a good substitute.

2 × 175g (2 × 6oz) fresh salmon fillets, skinned and boned
1 tsp vegetable bouillon stock powder
225g (8oz) [uncooked weight] pasta shapes
1 vegetable stock cube
300ml (½ pint) virtually fat free fromage frais
juice of ½ lemon
1 small red onion, finely chopped
1 tbsp chopped fresh chives
pinch of sweet paprika
fresh dill to garnish

1 Cook the salmon by poaching in a little water containing the stock powder for 8–10 minutes over a low heat. Lift the salmon from the pan and allow to cool.
2 Cook the pasta in a large saucepan of boiling water with the stock cube. Drain the pasta thoroughly and transfer to a mixing bowl. Add the fromage frais, lemon juice, onion, chives and paprika.
3 Carefully flake the salmon into the bowl, removing any bones and skin. Combine all the ingredients with a large metal spoon, taking care not to over-mix and break up the fish too much.

4 Spoon into a serving dish and chill until required. Garnish
   with fresh dill.

Creamy grilled lobster

SERVES 1
1 SERVING 228 KCAL/3.4G FAT
PREPARATION TIME 10 MINUTES
COOKING TIME 15 MINUTES

*Cooked lobsters are available in some supermarkets. Ask if they
can be split for you to save preparation time.*

1 cooked lobster (approx. 500g)
¼ tsp English mustard powder
¼ tsp cayenne pepper
1 tbsp chopped fresh chives
150ml (¼ pint) low-fat natural yogurt
25g (1oz) low-fat mature Cheddar cheese, grated
salt and freshly ground black pepper

1 Using a sharp knife, split the lobster in half lengthways by
   placing the point of the knife into the centre and pressing
   down through the shell. Remove the dark vein-like canal
   which runs along the length of the tail. Take out the meat
   from the main shell and place on a chopping board. Remove
   the stomach, which is under the head, and throw away.
   Throw away also the spongy material between the shell and
   the meat.
2 Chop the lobster meat and place in a small mixing bowl. You
   can add the liver, a soft creamy mass, to the meat.

3 Add the mustard, cayenne pepper, chives and yogurt. Season with salt and black pepper and mix the ingredients together. Carefully spoon the meat mixture back into the lobster shell and sprinkle with the cheese.

4 Place under a hot grill until golden brown and piping hot.

5 Just before serving, crack the claws, using lobster crackers or a rolling pin to make it easier to remove the claw meat. Serve hot.

Seafood pizza

SERVES 4
1 SERVING 389 KCAL/4.3G FAT
PREPARATION TIME 10 MINUTES
COOKING TIME 15 MINUTES

for the dough
225g (8oz) strong white bread flour
1 tsp salt
15g (½oz) fresh yeast or 2 tsps dried
150ml (¼ pint) warm skimmed milk

for the topping
300ml (½ pint) tomato passata
1 red pepper, seeded and finely chopped
1–2 fresh red chillies, sliced
1 tbsp chopped fresh oregano
450g (1lb) mixed cooked seafood (prawns, mussels, squid)
2 tbsps low-fat salad dressing
50g (2oz) low-fat Cheddar cheese, grated
a few basil leaves, shredded

1 Preheat the oven to 200C, 400F, Gas Mark 6.
2 Place the flour and salt into a large mixing bowl and make a slight well in the centre.
3 Dissolve the yeast in the milk, add to the flour and mix together with the blade of a round-ended knife, adding more liquid if required.
4 Turn out on to a floured surface and knead well to form a soft dough. Cover with a damp cloth for 10 minutes.
5 Knead the dough again. Divide into four equal parts. Roll out into four small circles and place on a non-stick baking tray.
6 For the topping, spoon the passata over the pizza bases, leaving a border around the edge of each one. Scatter with the red pepper, chillies and oregano and arrange the cooked seafood on top.
7 Mix together the salad dressing and the cheese and blob on top.
8 Bake the pizzas near the top of the oven for 10–15 minutes.
9 Just before serving scatter with the shredded basil. Serve hot.

Arrabbiata prawns

SERVES 4
1 SERVING 87 KCAL/0.7G FAT
PREPARATION TIME 20 MINUTES
COOKING TIME 30 MINUTES

225g (8oz) uncooked, peeled prawns
1 red onion, finely chopped
2 garlic cloves, crushed
1 red pepper, seeded and finely diced
1 × 400g can chopped tomatoes
1 red chilli, seeded and finely chopped
8–10 basil leaves
salt and freshly ground black pepper

1 Rinse the prawns well under cold, running water.
2 Preheat a non-stick frying pan. Add the onion and dry-fry
   for 2–3 minutes until soft.
3 Add the garlic and red pepper and cook for a further 2–3
   minutes.
4 Add the prawns and cook for 5–6 minutes.
5 Add the tomatoes and chilli, and bring the sauce to a gentle
   simmer. The prawns should be firm and cooked through.
6 Season to taste with salt and black pepper, add the basil
   leaves, and serve immediately.

Prawn and mushroom pasta

SERVES 4
1 SERVING 281 KCAL/2.6G FAT
PREPARATION TIME 20 MINUTES
COOKING TIME 30 MINUTES

225g (8oz) [uncooked weight] pasta shapes
1 vegetable stock cube
1 red onion, finely chopped
2 garlic cloves, crushed
1 red pepper, seeded and finely diced
115g (4oz) mushrooms, sliced
1 × 400g can chopped tomatoes
1 red chilli, finely sliced
2 × 160g packs cooked jumbo prawns
salt and freshly ground black pepper
1 tbsp finely chopped fresh chives to garnish

1 Cook the pasta in boiling salted water with vegetable stock
   cube.
2 Meanwhile, preheat a non-stick frying pan or wok. Add the
   onion and dry-fry for 2–3 minutes until soft. Add the garlic,
   red pepper and mushrooms and cook for a further 2–3
   minutes.
3 Add the tomatoes and chilli. Bring the sauce to a gentle
   simmer and add the prawns to heat through. Season to taste
   with salt and black pepper.
4 Drain the pasta and pour into a serving dish. Spoon the
   sauce over and sprinkle with the chives.

Prawn-fried rice

SERVES 4
1 SERVING 222 KCAL/2.3G FAT
PREPARATION TIME 20 MINUTES
COOKING TIME 10 MINUTES

1 large onion, finely chopped
2 garlic cloves, crushed
225g (8oz) cooked, peeled prawns
6 cardamom pods, crushed and seeds removed
½ tsp ground turmeric
1 small red chilli, finely chopped
150ml (¼ pint) vegetable stock
400g (14oz) [cooked weight] basmati rice
1 tbsp chopped fresh basil

1 Preheat a large wok or non-stick frying pan. Add the onion
   and garlic and dry-fry until soft.
2 Add the prawns and the spices and toss the ingredients well.
3 Pour in the stock and bring to the boil.
4 Add the rice and mix well until heated through.
5 Garnish with fresh basil before serving. Serve hot.

Vegetarian

Spicy chickpea burgers ⓥ

SERVES 4
1 SERVING 265 KCAL/73G FAT
PREPARATION TIME 20 MINUTES
COOKING TIME 10 MINUTES

Make these burgers in advance and refrigerate for 2 hours to allow them to hold together during cooking.

2 × 400g cans chickpeas
8 spring onions, chopped
1 garlic clove, crushed
1 tbsp finely chopped fresh ginger
2 tsps ground coriander
2 tsps garam masala
1 red chilli, finely chopped
1 egg, beaten
1–2 tsps vegetable stock powder
6–8 large basil leaves
freshly ground black pepper

1 Place all the ingredients in a food processor and blend, using a regular pulse motion, until coarsely chopped.
2 Scrape the mixture into a bowl and add plenty of freshly ground black pepper
3 Divide the mixture into four large balls. Using wet hands, mould into burger shapes by pressing the mixture well between both hands. Cover with food wrap and refrigerate until ready to use.

4 Cook the burgers under a hot grill for 5 minutes on each side until hot through to the centre.

Mexican bean bites with red pepper sauce Ⓥ

SERVES 4
1 SERVING 109 KCAL/3.4G FAT
PREPARATION TIME 20 MINUTES
COOKING TIME 10 MINUTES

1 red pepper
1 × 400g can red kidney beans, rinsed and drained
½ small red onion, chopped
1 garlic clove, crushed
2 tbsps chopped fresh coriander
½ –1 tbsp jalapeno chillies in brine, drained and chopped
½ × 200g can chopped tomatoes
¼ tsp smoked paprika
salt and freshly ground black pepper
sunflower oil spray (e.g. Fry Light)

1 Place the red pepper under a hot grill and cook, turning it, until blackened and blistered all over.
2 Meanwhile, put the beans in a food processor and blend for about 20 seconds or until chopped and chunky but not puréed. Tip into a bowl and fold in the onion, garlic, coriander and jalapenos and season with salt and black pepper. Mix well and then form into 24 balls. They can be refrigerated at this point.

3 Place the grilled pepper in a plastic bag to steam for 10 minutes. Remove the skin and seeds from the pepper, roughly chop the pepper and put into a food processor with the tomatoes and paprika and blend until smooth. Pour into a small pan, season with salt and black pepper, and heat gently.

4 Spray a large non-stick frying pan with a little sunflower oil spray, add the bean bites and warm for 3–4 minutes, rolling them gently over in the pan to heat through. Repeat if necessary with the remaining balls and serve with the sauce.

Moroccan chickpeas with spinach Ⓥ

SERVES 4
1 SERVING 218 KCAL/5G FAT
PREPARATION TIME 10 MINUTES
COOKING TIME 35 MINUTES

2 medium onions, chopped
1 tsp cumin seeds
2 garlic cloves, crushed
½ tsp ground ginger
½ tsp ground cinnamon
1 tsp ground coriander
30ml (1¼fl oz) vegetable stock
2 × 400g cans chickpeas, drained
4 ripe tomatoes, skinned and chopped
250g (10oz) spinach, washed
olive oil spray (e.g. Fry Light)
salt and freshly ground black pepper

1 Preheat a large frying pan or wok and spray with a little olive oil spray. Add the onions and cook for 5 minutes until browned. Stir in the cumin seeds and the garlic and cook for a further minute.

2 Add the remaining spices and mix well. Pour in the vegetable stock, bring to simmer then stir in the chickpeas and chopped tomatoes. Simmer, uncovered, for 20 minutes.

3 Meanwhile roughly shred the spinach, put into a large saucepan and cook for 2–3 minutes until wilted. Drain well through a sieve. Add to the chickpeas and cook for 2–3 minutes. Season with salt and black pepper, and serve.

Roasted Mediterranean tartlets Ⓥ

SERVES 6
1 SERVING 100 KCAL/1G FAT
PREPARATION TIME 15 MINUTES
COOKING TIME 30 MINUTES

1 aubergine
1 red and 1 yellow pepper, seeded
1 small red onion, peeled
2 courgettes, wiped
2 garlic cloves, finely chopped
2 sprigs of rosemary
1 tbsp balsamic vinegar
175g (6oz) cherry tomatoes, halved
3 sheets filo pastry
sunflower oil spray (e.g. Fry Light)
salt and freshly ground black pepper

1 Preheat the oven to 400F, 200C, Gas Mark 6.
2 Trim the aubergine and cut into dice. Cut the peppers into dice and the red onion into thin wedges. Trim and slice the courgettes. Place in a bowl and add the garlic, rosemary and balsamic vinegar. Season with salt and black pepper and toss well.
3 Transfer the vegetables to a non-stick baking tray and spray evenly with a little sunflower oil spray. Place in the oven and roast for 20 minutes. Add the cherry tomatoes and cook for a further 5 minutes.
4 Take a sheet of filo and spray with a little sunflower oil spray. Cut into six squares measuring approx. 10cm (4in) across. For each tartlet, use three squares of pastry. Ease the base squares into either Yorkshire pudding tins or tartlet tins. Place the remaining squares on top at different angles (the edges may need to be pushed in slightly to make an even-shaped case).
5 Line each tartlet with a little scrunched-up foil and bake for 8 minutes. Remove the foil and cook for a further 2–3 minutes until the pastry is golden and crispy.
6 Fill the tartlets with the roasted vegetables. Serve warm or cold.

Mixed pepper bruschetta ⓥ

SERVES 4
1 SERVING 166 KCAL/4.4G FAT
PREPARATION TIME 10 MINUTES
COOKING TIME 10 MINUTES

Make up these garlic toasts just before required and reheat in a low oven, as they will go soggy if left for more than 30 minutes.

⅓ French stick
2 garlic cloves
6 spring onions, finely chopped
1 small red and 1 small yellow pepper, seeded and finely diced
225g tomato passata
3–4 fresh basil leaves, finely shredded
4 cherry tomatoes, sliced
salt and freshly ground black pepper
salad leaves to garnish

1 Slice the bread diagonally into eight thick pieces and toast lightly under a hot grill on both sides. Slice 1 garlic clove in half. Rub both sides of the bread with the cut side and place on a baking tray.
2 Preheat a non-stick frying pan. Add the onions and dry-fry for 2–3 minutes until soft. Crush the remaining garlic clove and add to the pan along with the peppers. Cook until soft. Add the passata and simmer over a low heat until most of the moisture has evaporated to leave a paste-like consistency. Allow to cool, then stir in the basil and season to taste.

3 Spread the mixture on to the toasted bread and top with the
   sliced cherry tomatoes. Place under the hot grill to brown.
4 Garnish with the salad leaves and serve warm.

Penne with roasted vegetables Ⓥ

SERVES 4
1 SERVING 345 KCAL/3G FAT
PREPARATION TIME 15 MINUTES
COOKING TIME 40 MINUTES

1 medium aubergine, cut into chunks
3 medium courgettes, thickly sliced
3 red or yellow peppers, seeded and cut into chunks
1 tsp Italian dried herbs
250g (10oz) cherry tomatoes
1 × 400g can chopped tomatoes
1 or 2 garlic cloves, crushed
zest of ½ lemon
1 vegetable stock cube
300g (11oz) [uncooked weight] penne
1 vegetable stock cube
2 tbsps finely shredded basil
olive oil spray (e.g. Fry Light)
salt and freshly ground black pepper

1 Preheat the oven to 200C, 400F, Gas Mark 6.
2 Put the aubergine, courgettes and peppers into a large
   roasting tin, spray with a little olive oil spray to coat the
   vegetables, then season with salt and black pepper and scatter
   the dried herbs on top. With your hands, toss the vegetables
   together. Place in the oven to roast for 20 minutes.

3 Meanwhile put the cherry tomatoes and the chopped tomatoes into a small pan with the garlic and lemon zest and allow to simmer, uncovered, for 20 minutes until thick and pulpy.
4 Season the tomatoes with salt and black pepper, then add to the roasting tin and mix into the other vegetables. Return to the oven for 10 minutes.
5 Cook the penne in boiling water with the vegetable stock cube until al dente, then drain. Gently fold in the roasted vegetables and tomatoes. Sprinkle with basil and serve.

Spinach and leek pie ⓥ

SERVES 4
1 SERVING 257 KCAL/5G FAT
PREPARATION TIME 20–25 MINUTES
COOKING TIME 45 MINUTES

1 medium onion, chopped
50g (2oz) leeks, trimmed and chopped
1 vegetable stock cube
250g (10oz) spinach
1 tsp dried oregano
1 egg, beaten
1 × 250g carton low-fat cottage cheese
200g filo pastry
sunflower oil spray (e.g. Fry Light)
salt and freshly ground back pepper

1 Put the onion and leeks into a large pan. Stir the stock cube into 100ml (3½fl oz) hot water, and add to the pan. Cook over a medium heat, uncovered, for about 10 minutes until the vegetables are tender and the liquid has evaporated.

2 Meanwhile, trim the stalks from the spinach. Wash and shake off the excess water, then shred. Add to the pan and cook for 2 minutes until wilted. Tip into a colander and press out any excess liquid.

3 Preheat the oven to 200C, 400F, Gas Mark 6.

4 Put the vegetables into a bowl. Add the oregano, beaten egg and cottage cheese, season with salt and black pepper and mix well.

5 Spray a shallow rectangular tin (approx. 20 × 25cm/ 8 × 10in) with a little sunflower oil spray. Add a layer of filo pastry, allowing some pastry to hang over the edge. Spray with sunflower oil spray. Repeat three more layers of filo, spraying between each layer. Spoon the filling into the tin.

6 Top with three layers of filo pastry. Cut the pastry to fit within the tin but allow it to ruffle, and spray each layer. Fold in the overhanging pastry to make an edge and finally spray the folded edges.

7 Bake in the oven for about 30 minutes until golden. Cut into four portions and serve immediately.

Aubergine and mango kashmiri ⓥ ❄

SERVES 4
1 SERVING 246 KCAL/5.5G FAT
PREPARATION TIME 20 MINUTES
COOKING TIME 35 MINUTES

8 baby aubergines, cut in half (or 1 large aubergine, diced)
2 red onions, diced
2 garlic cloves, chopped
2 ripe mangoes, chopped
1–2 small red chillies, sliced
2 tsps ground turmeric
2 tsps tamarind paste
juice of 1 lime
1 × 2.5cm (1in) piece fresh ginger, peeled and chopped
4 kaffir lime leaves
1 × 410g can Carnation Light milk
8 cherry tomatoes
2 tbsps virtually fat free fromage frais
chopped fresh coriander to garnish

1 Preheat a non-stick pan. Add the aubergines, onions and
   garlic and dry-fry for 6–7 minutes until they start to colour.
2 Add the mangoes, chillies, turmeric and tamarind paste to
   the pan. Stir in the lime juice, ginger and kaffir lime leaves.
3 Stir in the milk and bring to the boil. Reduce the heat and
   simmer gently for 15–20 minutes until the vegetables are
   soft and the sauce has thickened.
4 When ready to serve, add the cherry tomatoes and allow to
   heat through.

5 Remove from the heat and stir in the fromage frais. Just before serving, sprinkle with chopped fresh coriander.

Cider and leek macaroni cheese ⓥ

SERVES 4
1 SERVING 369 KCAL/6.8G FAT
PREPARATION TIME 10 MINUTES
COOKING TIME 20 MINUTES

225g (8oz) [uncooked weight] macaroni
1 vegetable stock cube
6 baby leeks, trimmed and finely chopped
1 garlic clove, crushed
150ml (¼ pint) vegetable stock
1 tbsp plain flour
300ml (½ pint) skimmed milk
150ml (¼ pint) dry cider
115g (4oz) low-fat Cheddar cheese, grated
1 tsp Dijon mustard
salt and freshly ground black pepper
a few chopped chives to garnish

1 Cook the macaroni in a large pan of boiling water with the vegetable stock cube.
2 Preheat a non-stick pan. Add the leeks and garlic and dry-fry until soft. Add 2 tbsps of stock and stir in the flour. 'Cook out' the flour for 1 minute.
3 Gradually stir in the milk and remaining stock. Add the cider to the sauce along with the mustard and half the cheese. Season with salt and black pepper, reduce the heat and simmer for 2–3 minutes until the sauce thickens.

4 Drain the macaroni and pour into an ovenproof dish. Spoon the sauce over, and top with the remaining cheese.
5 Place under a medium hot grill to brown. Garnish with chopped chives before serving.

Vegetarian chilli Ⓥ ❄

SERVES 4
1 SERVING 206 KCAL/5G FAT (EXCLUDING NACHOS)
PREPARATION TIME 15 MINUTES
COOKING TIME 25 MINUTES

1 large red onion, chopped
2 garlic cloves, crushed
1 × 300g pack Quorn mince
2 × 400g cans chopped tomatoes
1 small red chilli, sliced
1–2 tsps chilli powder
300ml (½ pint) vegetable stock
1 × 400g can kidney beans, drained and rinsed
salt and freshly ground black pepper
low-fat yogurt to garnish
Oven-Baked Nachos (see recipe, page 245) to serve

1 Preheat a non-stick frying pan or wok. Add the onion and garlic and dry-fry until soft.
2 Add the Quorn mince and continue cooking over a high heat. Add the tomatoes, chilli, chilli powder, stock and kidney beans, season with salt and pepper, and bring the sauce to a gentle simmer.
3 Allow to simmer for 15 minutes, then spoon into a serving dish. Garnish with low-fat yogurt and serve with the nachos.

Vegetable quiche ⓥ

SERVES 4
1 SERVING 235 KCAL/3.6G FAT
PREPARATION TIME 30 MINUTES
COOKING TIME 40–45 MINUTES

450g (1lb) potatoes, peeled and cut into even-sized pieces
1–2 tbsps skimmed or semi-skimmed milk
2 tbsps flour
350g (12oz) carrots, sliced
2 tbsps low-fat fromage frais
1 egg
pinch of nutmeg
175g (6oz) mushrooms, trimmed and sliced
3 medium tomatoes, sliced
2–3 tsps fresh breadcrumbs
2 tsps grated Parmesan cheese
salt and freshly ground black pepper

1 Preheat the oven to 200C, 400F, Gas Mark 6
2 Cook the potatoes in boiling salted water until tender. Drain
   well and mash until smooth with the milk and flour. Season
   with salt and black pepper.
3 Place in the bottom of a 18cm (7in) quiche dish. Press out
   with a spoon to fill the bottom of the dish evenly.
4 Cook the carrots in boiling salted water until tender. Drain
   well and place in a blender with the fromage frais and the
   egg. Season to taste with salt, black pepper and nutmeg.
   Pour into the potato case.
5 Place the sliced mushrooms and tomatoes in layers over the
   carrot mixture.

6 Mix together the breadcrumbs and Parmesan. Season lightly and sprinkle over the vegetables.
7 Bake in the oven until the potato is golden and the mushrooms are cooked. Serve hot.

Baked cheesy sweet potatoes ⓥ

SERVES 4
1 SERVING 267 KCAL/5G FAT
PREPARATION TIME 10 MINUTES
COOKING TIME 1 HOUR

4 large sweet potatoes
2 tbsps half-fat crème fraîche
2 tbsps grated low-fat Cheddar cheese
1 tbsp chopped fresh chives
coarse sea salt

1 Preheat the oven to 200C, 400F, Gas Mark 6.
2 Scrub the sweet potatoes and place in a non-stick roasting tin.
3 Sprinkle with sea salt and place in the oven for approximately 1 hour, until cooked.
4 When cooked, remove from the oven and cut in half. Combine the crème fraîche, cheese and chives in a small bowl. Spoon into the centre of each potato and return to the oven for a further 10 minutes until the cheese has melted. Serve hot.

Lentil salad Ⓥ

SERVES 2
1 SERVING 262 KCAL/8G FAT
PREPARATION TIME 1½ HOURS
COOKING TIME 35–50 MINUTES

This can be served as an accompaniment to a main course or as a light lunch. If you don't have time to cook the lentils, you can use canned ones instead.

1 onion, sliced
2 celery sticks, sliced
2 garlic cloves, crushed
175g (6oz) [uncooked weight] brown or green lentils, soaked
    for at least 1½ hours
1 × 400g can black-eyed beans, rinsed and drained
½ each red, green and yellow peppers, seeded and diced
115g (4oz) cucumber, diced
6 tbsps reduced-fat salad dressing
25g (1oz) Parmesan shavings
sunflower spray oil (e.g. Fry Light)

1 Spray a saucepan with sunflower spray oil. Add the onion, celery and garlic and cook for 5 minutes until softened.
2 Add the lentils and 300ml (½ pint) boiling water. Cover and simmer gently for 30–45 minutes until the lentils are tender. Drain if necessary and allow to cool.
3 When cold, stir in the beans, peppers and cucumber. Add the dressing and toss well. Sprinkle with the Parmesan shavings.

Fresh tomato and basil pasta Ⓥ

SERVES 2
1 SERVING 366 KCAL/1.7G FAT
PREPARATION TIME 20 MINUTES
COOKING TIME 30 MINUTES

175g (6oz) [uncooked weight] pasta shapes
1 vegetable stock cube
75g (3oz) fresh basil leaves
1 garlic clove, crushed
1 tsp vegetable stock powder
225g (8oz) cherry tomatoes, cut in half
2 tbsps virtually fat free fromage frais
25g (1oz) freshly grated Parmesan
salt and freshly ground black pepper

1 Cook the pasta in boiling salted water with the vegetable
  stock cube.
2 Meanwhile pick the basil leaves from the stems and place in
  a food processor. Add the garlic, stock powder and 2 tbsps
  boiling water and process until smooth.
3 Drain the pasta and pour back into the saucepan. Add the
  basil pesto, fromage frais and cherry tomatoes. Mix well and
  season with salt and black pepper.
4 Pile into a serving dish and finish with a little freshly grated
  Parmesan cheese if desired.

Parsnip and chestnut herb roast ⓥ ❄

SERVES 6
1 SERVING 235 KCAL/5G FAT
PREPARATION TIME 20 MINUTES
COOKING TIME 1 HOUR

225g (8oz) parsnips
1 onion, finely chopped
1 garlic clove, crushed
1 × 435g can chestnut purée
115g (4oz) [uncooked weight] red lentils
1 × 400g can chopped tomatoes
300ml (½ pint) vegetable stock
2 tsps finely chopped mixed herbs
2 eggs, beaten
grated fresh nutmeg
salt and freshly ground black pepper

1 Preheat the oven to 150C, 300F, Gas Mark 2.
2 Peel the parsnips and cut into dice. Place in a small
   saucepan. Cover with water and cook until soft.
3 Preheat a non-stick frying pan or wok. Add the onion and
   garlic and cook until soft.
4 Add the chestnut purée, lentils, chopped tomatoes and
   vegetable stock. Simmer gently for 10 minutes until the
   lentils are soft and some of the liquid has evaporated.
   Remove from the heat and pour into a mixing bowl.
5 Stir the cooked parsnips and the herbs into the lentil
   mixture. Pour in the beaten eggs and mix well. Season with
   salt, black pepper and nutmeg.

6 Pour the mixture into a lightly greased 1kg (2lb) loaf tin. Bake in the oven for 1 hour until firm to touch. Allow to cool slightly before turning out.
7 When cool, cut into slices, place on a baking tray and cover with foil. Place in a low oven for 10 minutes to reheat.

Roasted butternut squash and tomato tart Ⓥ

SERVES 6
1 SERVING 185 KCAL/5.9G FAT
PREPARATION TIME 40 MINUTES
COOKING TIME 20 MINUTES

1 medium butternut squash
2 garlic cloves, sliced
1 tbsp light soy sauce
6 sheets filo pastry
1 egg white, beaten
1 tbsp fresh thyme leaves
2 tsps vegetable bouillon stock powder
115g (4oz) low-fat Cheddar cheese
2 eggs, beaten
8 cherry tomatoes
1 tbsp chopped fresh chives
salt and freshly ground black pepper

1 Preheat the oven to 190C, 375F, Gas Mark 5.
2 Peel, seed and roughly dice the squash and place in the base of a baking tray. Cover with the garlic and drizzle with soy sauce. Bake in the top of the oven for 20 minutes or until soft.

3 Lightly grease a 23cm (9in) flan tin. Unfold the filo pastry. Taking a sheet at a time, lightly brush with egg white and place in the base of the tin. Continue placing the other sheets on top, tucking the edges into the sides of the tin and brushing each sheet with egg white.

4 Bake in the oven for 4–5 minutes until dry. Allow to cool.

5 Place the roasted squash and garlic in a mixing bowl. Add the thyme, stock powder, cheese and eggs and mix together, seasoning to taste. Spoon into the pastry case and arrange the tomatoes on top. Scatter the chives over.

6 Bake in the oven for 15–20 minutes until set. Serve warm.

Asparagus and vegetable bake ⓥ

SERVES 4
1 SERVING 466 KCAL/10G FAT
PREPARATION TIME 15 MINUTES
COOKING TIME 35 MINUTES

225g (8oz) baby carrots, chopped
225g (8oz) baby parsnips, chopped
1 vegetable stock cube
115g (4oz) baby leeks, trimmed and chopped
115g (4oz) broccoli florets
2 large courgettes, sliced
1 large bunch baby asparagus
600ml (1 pint) skimmed milk
1 tbsp wholegrain mustard
1 tbsp cornflour
115g (4oz) low-fat Cheddar cheese
2 tbsps chopped fresh chives

1 Preheat the oven to 190C, 375F, Gas Mark 5.
2 Place the carrots and parsnips in a small saucepan. Cover
   with water, bring to the boil, add the stock cube and cook for
   4 minutes. Add the leeks, broccoli, courgettes and asparagus
   and simmer for a further 2–3 minutes until the broccoli is just
   cooked.
3 Remove from the heat, drain through a colander and place in
   the bottom of an ovenproof dish.
4 Add the milk and the mustard to the pan and heat. Slake the
   cornflour with a little cold water and mix into the milk. Bring
   to the boil, stirring continuously. Remove from the heat and
   stir in the cheese and chives.
4 Pour the sauce over the vegetables and place in the oven for
   20 minutes until golden brown.

Spinach and ricotta cannelloni Ⓥ ❄

SERVES 4
1 SERVING 422 KCAL/11G FAT
PREPARATION TIME 10 MINUTES
COOKING TIME 40 MINUTES

225g (8oz) fresh spinach
225g (8oz) ricotta cheese
225g (8oz) Quark (low-fat soft cheese)
2 garlic cloves, crushed
225g (8oz) tomato passata
1 tbsp chopped fresh oregano
16 cannelloni tubes
salt and freshly ground black pepper

for the topping
600ml (1 pint) skimmed milk
2 tsps vegetable stock powder
1 tsp English mustard powder
1 tbsp cornflour
1 tbsp white wine
salt and freshly ground black pepper
2 tsps freshly grated Parmesan

1 Preheat the oven to 200C, 400F, Gas Mark 6.
2 Using a large chopping knife, finely chop the spinach and place in a mixing bowl. Add the ricotta, Quark and garlic and mix well, seasoning with lots of salt and black pepper.
3 Pour the passata into the bottom of a rectangular ovenproof dish and sprinkle with the chopped oregano.
4 Place the spinach mixture into a piping bag without a nozzle and pipe the filling into the cannelloni tubes. Place the filled pasta on top of the passata.
5 To make the topping, heat the milk, stock powder and mustard in a saucepan to near boiling. Slake the cornflour with the wine and whisk into the hot milk. Season with black pepper and simmer gently to allow the sauce to thicken.
6 Pour the sauce over the pasta and place in the oven for 30 minutes. Sprinkle with the Parmesan and serve hot.

Lentil roast ⓥ

SERVES 4
1 SERVING 377 KCAL/1.9G FAT
PREPARATION TIME 20 MINUTES
COOKING TIME 1 HOUR

350g (12oz) [uncooked weight] orange lentils
1 bay leaf
2–3 parsley stalks
1 sprig fresh thyme
2 large onions, chopped
1–2 garlic cloves, crushed
1 tsp ground cumin
2–3 celery sticks, sliced
1 vegetable stock cube
1 eating apple
½ green pepper, seeded and diced
½ red pepper, seeded and diced
1 × 400g can chopped tomatoes
75g (3oz) Quark or low-fat natural yogurt
salt and freshly ground black pepper

1 Preheat the oven to 180C, 350F, Gas Mark 4.
2 Wash the lentils well, drain and place in a large pan. Cover
  with water.
3 Tie the bay leaf, parsley stalks and thyme together with
  string and add to the pan. Bring to the boil.
4 Add the onions, garlic, cumin and celery to the lentils, along
  with the stock cube, and simmer until the lentils and
  vegetables are tender and the liquid has almost evaporated.

5 Meanwhile, peel the apple, cut into quarters and remove the core. Cut the quarters into small dice.
6 When the lentils are tender, remove the bunch of herbs and continue cooking, stirring all the time until the mixture is quite dry.
7 Stir the diced apple, peppers, tomatoes and Quark or yogurt into the lentil mixture. Mix well and season to taste with salt and black pepper.
8 Pile the mixture into an ovenproof dish and bake in the oven for about 1 hour, until the top is springy like a sponge. Serve hot or cold.

Sweet potato, pepper and fennel bake ⓥ

SERVES 4
1 SERVING 340 KCAL/4G FAT
PREPARATION TIME 30 MINUTES
COOKING TIME 55 MINUTES

675g (1½lb) sweet potatoes, diced
1 large bulb fennel, thinly sliced
2 red peppers, seeded and finely sliced
4 leeks, trimmed, washed and sliced
2 garlic cloves, crushed
600ml (1 pint) skimmed milk
2 tsps vegetable bouillon powder
2 tbsps cornflour
50g (2oz) low-fat Cheddar cheese
2 tbsps chopped fresh chives
salt and freshly ground black pepper

1 Preheat the oven to 200C, 400F, Gas Mark 6.
2 Cook the sweet potatoes in boiling, salted water. Drain well.
3 Preheat a non-stick pan. Add the fennel and dry-fry until it starts to colour. Remove from the pan and set aside.
4 Add the peppers, leeks and garlic to the pan and cook over a high heat until they start to colour.
5 Heat the milk and stock powder in a saucepan until boiling. Slake the cornflour with a little water and add to the milk, stirring continuously to prevent any lumps forming.
6 Mix in the cheese and chives and season with salt and black pepper.
7 In an ovenproof dish place alternate layers of sweet potato, fennel sauce and vegetable mixture, finishing with a layer of potato.
8 Bake in the oven for 20–25 minutes until brown and crisp.

Stir-fry Quorn ⓥ

SERVES 4
1 SERVING 130 KCAL/4.8G FAT
PREPARATION TIME 15 MINUTES
COOKING TIME 10 MINUTES

450g (1lb) Quorn chunks
2 tsps ground coriander
8 spring onions, chopped
115g (4oz) pak choi or spring greens
115g (4oz) mangetout
2 medium carrots, cut into julienne strips
grated root ginger to taste
1–2 tsps soy sauce
juice of 1 lemon
olive oil spray (e.g. Fry Light)
salt and freshly ground black pepper

1 Spray a non-stick wok or pan lightly with olive oil spray. Add
  the Quorn, ground coriander and spring onions and cook for
  a few minutes.
2 Add the remaining vegetables and the grated ginger.
  Continue to cook until the Quorn and vegetables are cooked
  but the vegetables are still crunchy.
3 Add the soy sauce and lemon juice. Season with salt and
  black pepper and serve immediately.

Tofu noodle stir-fry ⓥ

SERVES 4
1 SERVING 317 KCAL/6.5G FAT
PREPARATION TIME 20 MINUTES
COOKING TIME 10 MINUTES

225g (8oz) tofu
2 long shallots, peeled and sliced
2 orange peppers, seeded and sliced
1 × 2.5cm (1in) piece fresh ginger, finely chopped
225g (8oz) pack baby corn, carrots and mangetout
225g (8oz) beansprouts
225g (8oz) straight-to-wok noodles
1 tbsp light soy sauce
olive oil spray (e.g. Fry Light)
salt and freshly ground black pepper
chopped fresh chives to garnish

1 Drain the tofu well and pat dry with kitchen paper. Cut into pieces and season with salt and black pepper.
2 Heat a non-stick wok or pan until hot. Lightly spray with olive oil spray and add the tofu. Cook quickly over a high heat, tossing the tofu pieces so that they brown evenly. Remove from the pan and place on a plate.
3 Return the pan to the heat, add the shallots and peppers, and cook over a high heat. Add the ginger and corn and carrots, tossing them well. Add the mangetout and beansprouts and mix well for 2 minutes. Fold in the noodles and soy sauce until completely heated through. Return the tofu to the pan and stir well.
4 Pile into a serving dish and sprinkle with chopped chives.

Aubergine and spinach pasta bake ⓥ ❄

SERVES 4
1 SERVING 300 KCAL/6.6G FAT
PREPARATION TIME 10 MINUTES
COOKING TIME 30 MINUTES

175g (6oz) [uncooked weight] rigatoni pasta
2 vegetable stock cubes
225g (8oz) young spinach leaves, shredded
1 red onion, finely chopped
1 aubergine, diced
2 garlic cloves, crushed
1 red pepper, seeded and finely chopped
1 × 400g can chopped tomatoes
1 red chilli, seeded and finely chopped
8–10 basil leaves, shredded
115g (4oz) low-fat Cheddar cheese, grated
salt and freshly ground black pepper

1 Preheat the oven to 190C, 375F, Gas Mark 5.
2 Cook the pasta in plenty of boiling water with 1 vegetable
  stock cube until al dente. Drain well, and stir in the shredded
  spinach leaves.
3 Meanwhile, preheat a non-stick frying pan or wok. Add the
  red onion and dry-fry for 2–3 minutes until soft. Add the
  aubergine, garlic and red pepper and cook for a further 6–8
  minutes until the aubergine starts to colour.
4 Add the tomatoes, chilli and remaining stock cube and bring
  the sauce to a gentle simmer. Season to taste with salt and
  black pepper.

5 Pour the pasta into a large ovenproof serving dish. Cover with the sauce and then sprinkle with the shredded basil leaves and grated Cheddar cheese.

6 Bake in the oven for about 15–20 minutes until golden brown on top.

Lemon and mustard seed humous Ⓥ

SERVES 4
1 SERVING 148 KCAL/4.7G FAT
PREPARATION TIME 10 MINUTES
COOKING TIME 15 MINUTES

1 × 425g can chickpeas with no added salt or sugar
300ml (½ pint) soya milk
2 garlic cloves, crushed
2 tsps mustard seed
juice of 1 lemon
salt
cayenne pepper to taste

1 Drain and rinse the chickpeas and place in a food processor.

2 Pour in the milk, garlic and mustard seed and process until smooth. Season with salt and pepper, add the lemon juice, then blend again to combine. Adjust the consistency with a little extra milk if required and adjust the seasoning to taste.

Side dishes and accompaniments

Oven-baked nachos ⓥ

SERVES 4
1 SERVING 128 KCAL/2.5G FAT
PREPARATION TIME 5 MINUTES
COOKING TIME 20 MINUTES

These crunchy nibbles make a tasty low-fat alternative to crisps.

4 corn tortillas

1 Preheat the oven to 150C, 300F, Gas Mark 2.
2 Place the tortillas on a chopping board. Using a heavy chopping knife, cut each one in half. Cut the halves into quarters and place on a non-stick baking tray.
3 Bake in the centre of the oven for 20 minutes. Remove from the oven and allow to cool and crisp up.

Roasted red pepper couscous ⓥ

SERVES 2
1 SERVING 96 KCAL/0.6G FAT
PREPARATION TIME 20 MINUTES
COOKING TIME 5 MINUTES

This sweet-flavoured accompaniment can be made in advance and stored in the refrigerator. Reheat by steaming over a pan of boiling water or simply cover with foil in a moderate oven.

1 large red pepper
50g (2oz) [uncooked weight] couscous
1 tsp vegetable bouillon powder
1 tsp ground coriander
1 tbsp finely chopped fresh chives
1 tbsp chopped fresh coriander
salt and freshly ground black pepper

1 Preheat the oven to 200C, 400F, Gas Mark 6.
2 Place the red pepper on a baking tray and roast uncovered
   for 15–20 minutes until soft. Remove from oven and place
   immediately into a plastic food bag and seal. Allow to cool
   completely then remove from the bag and peel away the
   skin. Slice the pepper in half and remove the seeds. Chop the
   flesh into dice and set aside.
3 Measure the couscous in a cup. Place the same amount of
   water in a saucepan and bring to the boil.
4 Add the bouillon powder and coriander and gradually pour in
   the couscous, stirring well. Cover with a lid, remove from the
   heat and allow to stand for 1 minute.
5 Remove the lid and, using two forks, fluff up the couscous
   grains. Add the herbs, mix well and season to taste. Add the
   chopped pepper and arrange on serving plates.

Roast sweet potatoes with chilli glaze Ⓥ

SERVES 4
1 SERVING 124 KCAL/0.5G FAT
PREPARATION TIME 10 MINUTES
COOKING TIME 35 MINUTES

450g (1lb) sweet potatoes
1 vegetable stock cube
1 medium red onion, finely diced
2 tbsps light soy sauce
1 tsp sea salt
1 red chilli, seeded and finely chopped
1 garlic clove, crushed
2 tbsps apple sauce
1 tbsp chopped fresh parsley

1 Preheat the oven to 200C, 400F, Gas Mark 6.
2 Wash the potatoes and cut into 2.5cm (1in) pieces. Cook in a
   pan of boiling water with the vegetable stock cube for 5
   minutes, then drain well.
3 Place the potatoes in the bottom of a non-stick baking tin.
   Add the red onion. Drizzle the soy sauce over and sprinkle
   with a little sea salt. Bake in the oven for 20–25 minutes.
4 Remove from the oven. Combine the chilli, garlic and apple
   sauce and dot over the potatoes. Shake the tin well to coat
   the potatoes then return to the oven for 5 minutes. Just
   before serving sprinkle with parsley.

Ratatouille mushrooms Ⓥ

SERVES 2
1 SERVING 148 KCAL/1.4G FAT
PREPARATION TIME 10 MINUTES
COOKING TIME 25 MINUTES

4 large open mushrooms
2 medium onions, sliced
225g (8oz) courgettes, sliced
1 small aubergine, sliced
1 large red pepper, seeded and finely sliced
1 × 400g can chopped tomatoes
2 garlic cloves, crushed
2 tsps chopped fresh thyme
olive oil spray (e.g. Fry Light)
salt and freshly ground black pepper
fresh basil to garnish

1 Place the mushrooms on a baking tray and lightly spray with
   olive oil spray. Place under a hot grill and cook for 3–4
   minutes on each side.
2 Preheat a non-stick frying pan or wok. Add the onions and
   dry-fry until soft. Add the courgettes, season with salt and
   black pepper, and cook for a further 2–3 minutes. Pour into a
   saucepan.
3 Add the aubergine and red pepper to the frying pan, season
   and dry-fry for 4–5 minutes. Transfer to the saucepan.
4 Pour the tomatoes into the frying pan, add the garlic, and
   thyme, bring to the boil, and then pour over the vegetables.
5 Place the saucepan on the heat and simmer for 10 minutes.

6 Spoon the vegetables on to the mushrooms. Just before
   serving, sprinkle with fresh basil.

Garlic and herb roasted potatoes ⓥ ❄

SERVES 4
1 SERVING 89 KCAL/0.4G FAT
PREPARATION TIME 15 MINUTES
COOKING TIME 45 MINUTES

450g (1lb) charlotte potatoes
8 garlic cloves with skin intact
2–3 sprigs fresh rosemary
2–3 sprigs fresh thyme
2 tbsps light soy sauce
chopped fresh flat-leaf parsley to garnish
salt

1 Preheat the oven to 200C, 400F, Gas Mark 6.
2 Cook the potatoes in lightly salted boiling water. Drain and
   place in a non-stick roasting tin.
3 Dot the garlic and herbs over the potatoes, pulling the herb
   leaves away from the stems. Drizzle with soy sauce and toss
   the potatoes to coat them with the mixture.
4 Place in the oven and roast for 35–45 minutes, shaking the
   pan occasionally to prevent sticking.
5 Transfer to a serving bowl and garnish with parsley.

Stir-fried mushrooms and peppers Ⓥ

SERVES 4
1 SERVING 46 KCAL/0.7G FAT
PREPARATION TIME 20 MINUTES
COOKING TIME 10 MINUTES

For added flavour add 1–2 crushed garlic cloves to the pan during cooking.

2 red and 2 yellow peppers, seeded and diced
225g (8oz) button mushrooms, rinsed
zest and juice of 1 lemon
1 tbsp light soy sauce
1 tbsp chopped fresh chives

1 Place the diced peppers in a bowl. Add the mushrooms, pour the lemon zest and juice and the soy sauce over and toss well to coat the vegetables.
2 Preheat a non-stick wok or pan. Add the vegetables and cook quickly over a high heat, tossing them so that they cook evenly.
3 Pile into a serving dish and sprinkle with chopped chives.

Griddled asparagus with fresh lemon and cracked black pepper Ⓥ

SERVES 4
1 SERVING 88 KCAL/3.4G FAT
PREPARATION TIME 15 MINUTES
COOKING TIME 15 MINUTES

2 bunches (1kg/2lb) fairly thick fresh asparagus
1 vegetable stock cube
1 lemon, cut into quarters
1 tsp cracked black pepper
2 tbsps Parmesan shavings

1 Trim or break the asparagus stems off. Using a vegetable peeler, shave away 5cm (2in) from the base of each stem. Blanch by placing in a pan of boiling water with the vegetable stock cube, and cook for 3–4 minutes.
2 Drain the asparagus (you can retain the cooking water to use in soup and sauces).
3 Preheat a griddle pan until hot. Add the asparagus and cook for 2–3 minutes on each side until slightly charred. Squeeze the lemon juice over and season with cracked black pepper.
4 Serve hot, sprinkled with a few Parmesan shavings.

Baked winter vegetables ⓥ

SERVES 4
1 SERVING 160 KCAL/1.7G FAT
PREPARATION TIME 10 MINUTES
COOKING TIME 40 MINUTES

1kg (2lb) pumpkin or gourd, peeled and seeded
450g (1lb) baby beetroot, washed
450g (1lb) carrots, washed
450g (1lb) celeriac, peeled
450g (1lb) swede, peeled
6 garlic cloves
olive oil spray (e.g. Fry Light)
salt and freshly ground black pepper
chopped fresh chives to garnish

1 Preheat the oven to 180C, 350F, Gas Mark 4.
2 Cut the vegetables into bite-sized pieces and place in a non-stick roasting tin. Season with salt and black pepper.
3 Using the broad edge of a chopping knife, crush the garlic cloves against a chopping board and add to the vegetables.
4 Spray the vegetables lightly with olive oil spray and mix well.
5 Roast, uncovered, in the oven for 40 minutes until tender.
6 Just before serving sprinkle with chives.

Sautéed courgettes and cherry tomatoes Ⓥ

SERVES 4
1 SERVING 22 KCAL/0.5G FAT
PREPARATION TIME 10 MINUTES
COOKING TIME 20 MINUTES

Choose small young courgettes with a shiny bloom. Old courgettes become tough and withered and have a strong, bitter flavour.

225g (8oz) courgettes, sliced
1 garlic clove, crushed
pinch of sea salt
225g (8oz) cherry tomatoes, cut in half
freshly ground black pepper
a few basil leaves to garnish

1 Preheat a non-stick frying pan or wok. Add the courgettes and garlic and dry-fry over a moderate heat for 5–6 minutes until soft. Season with salt and black pepper.
2 Add the tomatoes and continue cooking for 1–2 minutes to heat through. Just before serving sprinkle with fresh basil.

Garlic mushrooms ⓥ

SERVES 4
1 SERVING 74 KCAL/4G FAT
PREPARATION TIME 5 MINUTES
COOKING TIME 15 MINUTES

225g (1oz) (8oz) baby button mushrooms, wiped
225g (1oz) (8oz) open cap mushrooms, wiped and sliced
150g (5oz) shiitake mushrooms, wiped and halved
1 tsp medium sherry
1 tsp soy sauce
Fry Light garlic spray

for the topping
25g (1oz) fresh white breadcrumbs
25g (1oz) freshly grated Parmesan cheese

1 Preheat a large non-stick frying pan and spray with a little
  Fry Light garlic. Add the prepared mushrooms and stir-fry for
  5 minutes.
2 Add the sherry and soy sauce to the pan, toss thoroughly
  and cook for a further 2–3 minutes.
3 Spoon the cooked mushrooms into four individual serving
  dishes.
4 For the topping, mix together the breadcrumbs and
  Parmesan and scatter over each dish. Spray the top of each
  one with a little Fry Light garlic and place under a medium
  hot grill for 3–4 minutes, until golden and crispy. Serve
  immediately.

Fried carrots and green chillies ⓥ

SERVES 4
1 SERVING 59 KCAL/0.6G FAT
PREPARATION TIME 10 MINUTES
COOKING TIME 10 MINUTES

450g (1lb) carrots, coarsely grated
1 red onion, sliced
2 small green chillies, sliced
pinch of stock powder
1 tsp cumin seed
1 tsp ground coriander
zest and juice of 1 lime

1 Using the coarse side of a cheese grater, grate the carrot into a large mixing bowl. Add the onion along with the remaining ingredients and mix well.
2 Preheat a wok or non-stick deep-sided frying pan. Add the carrot mixture and cook quickly over a high heat for 5–6 minutes, tossing well.
3 Serve hot as a vegetable accompaniment or cold as a spicy salad.

Minted cucumber and red onion salad Ⓥ

SERVES 4
1 SERVING 49 KCAL/0.2G FAT
PREPARATION TIME 10 MINUTES

This simple side dish takes only minutes to prepare. If made in advance, drain before serving, as the cucumber will release water once stood.

2 cucumbers
2 red onions
2 tbsps chopped fresh mint
2 tbsps fruit vinegar
2 oranges
salt and freshly ground black pepper

1 Using the coarse side of a grater, grate both the cucumbers and the red onions into a bowl. Add the mint and vinegar and season well with salt and black pepper.
2 Using a serrated knife, cut away the peel from the oranges and segment the fruit over the bowl to catch any juice.
3 Mix well and spoon into a serving dish. Serve straight away.

Spanish salad

SERVES 4
1 SERVING 119 KCAL/4.5G FAT
PREPARATION TIME 15 MINUTES

2 romaine lettuce
4 tomatoes
50g (2oz) white anchovy fillets, rinsed and cut in half
115g (4oz) peeled, cooked prawns
8 guindilla chillies
8 stuffed green olives, sliced

for the lemon dressing
4 tbsps lemon juice
2 tbsps fresh apple juice
1 tbsp honey
2 tbsps Dijon mustard

1 Wash the lettuce, drain well and tear into small pieces. Place
   in salad bowl.
2 Peel and quarter the tomatoes and remove the seeds. Add to
   the lettuce. Add the anchovies, prawns, guindilla chillies and
   olives.
3 To make the lemon dressing, place all the ingredients into a
   bowl and stir well, then pour over the salad and toss lightly.
   Serve immediately.

Crunchy green Gi salad Ⓥ

SERVES 1
1 SERVING 54 KCAL/0.09G FAT
PREPARATION TIME 15 MINUTES

50g (2oz) salad leaves of your choice, shredded
½ green pepper, seeded and chopped
1 × 2.5cm (1in) chunk cucumber, chopped
4 spring onions, chopped
2 celery sticks, finely chopped
4 basil leaves left whole (optional)
5 fresh mangetout or sugar snap peas, coarsely chopped
1 tbsp oil-free dressing

1 Place all the ingredients in a bowl and mix well.
2 Add oil-free dressing to taste and toss well.

Sweet and sour cucumber Ⓥ

SERVES 4
1 SERVING 58 KCAL/0.4G FAT
PREPARATION TIME 10 MINUTES
COOKING TIME 10 MINUTES

1 cucumber
1 × 250g can pineapple pieces
1 × 200g pack beansprouts
2 tbsps sweet chilli sauce
1 tbsp rice wine vinegar
salt and freshly ground black pepper

1 Top and tail the cucumber and cut into slices.
2 Preheat a non-stick wok, add the cucumber and cook over a high heat for 2–3 minutes.
3 Add the remaining ingredients and toss well. Continue cooking until the beansprouts start to wilt. Pile into a serving dish and serve straight away.

Sweet potato and cucumber salad Ⓥ

SERVES 4
1 SERVING 145 KCAL 0.9G FAT
PREPARATION TIME 10 MINUTES

450g (1lb) sweet potatoes
1 cucumber
2 red onions, finely chopped
2 tbsps chopped fresh flat-leaf parsley
2 tbsps fruit vinegar
2 tsps Dijon or grain mustard
1 tsp runny honey
salt and freshly ground black pepper

1 Using the coarse side of a grater, grate both the sweet potatoes and cucumber into a bowl. Add the onions and parsley. Mix well and season with salt and freshly ground black pepper.
2 Combine the vinegar, mustard and honey in a small bowl. Using a balloon whisk, mix the ingredients together until fully combined.
3 Pour the dressing over the salad and pile into a serving dish.

Tomato, spinach and balsamic onion salad ⓥ

SERVES 4
1 SERVING 59 KCAL/1.3G FAT
PREPARATION TIME 15 MINUTES
COOKING TIME 10 MINUTES

1 red onion, finely sliced
1 tsp lemon thyme
2 tbsps good-quality balsamic vinegar
4 ripe vine tomatoes
225g (8oz) young baby spinach or ruby chard

for the dressing
150ml (¼ pint) vegetable stock
2 good handfuls fresh basil
1 garlic clove, crushed
1 tbsp cooked chestnuts, peeled and finely chopped
salt and freshly ground black pepper

1 Preheat a non-stick frying pan or wok. Add the onion and dry-fry for 2–3 minutes until soft. Add the thyme and balsamic vinegar and allow to cool.
2 Place all the dressing ingredients in a blender or food processor and blend until smooth.
3 Assemble the salad by mixing the tomatoes, spinach and balsamic onions together. Serve the dressing separately.

Orange and fennel Greek salad Ⓥ

SERVES 4
1 SERVING 82 KCAL/0.5G FAT
PREPARATION TIME 10 MINUTES
COOKING TIME 20 MINUTES

2 small heads fennel, finely sliced
2 large oranges, peeled and segmented
2 tbsps fruit vinegar
115g (4oz) Quark low-fat soft cheese
1 garlic clove, crushed
1 tbsp chopped fresh basil
1 romaine or crisp lettuce
½ cucumber, peeled and diced
1 small red onion, finely sliced
2 beef tomatoes, cut into chunks
a few black grapes
salt and freshly ground black pepper
chopped fresh flat-leaf parsley to garnish

1 Place the fennel in a bowl with the oranges and the fruit
   vinegar.
2 Mix together the Quark, garlic and basil, and season with salt
   and pepper. Using a teaspoon, take small amounts of the
   cheese mixture and roll into balls.
3 Arrange the salad leaves on a serving plate. Add the
   cucumber, onion, tomato and grapes.
4 Arrange the cheese balls on the leaves and spoon the
   marinated fennel and oranges on top. Sprinkle with parsley
   and serve.

Desserts

Blueberry syllabub

SERVES 4
1 SERVING 103 KCAL/0.7G FAT
PREPARATION TIME 10 MINUTES
COOKING TIME 15 MINUTES

Choose a creamy low-fat yogurt for a smoother, luxurious finish.

225g (8oz) blueberries
1 tbsp Madeira wine
2 tbsps golden caster sugar
zest and juice of 1 lime
225g (8oz) low-fat Greek yogurt
2 tsps Amaretto liqueur
1 fresh egg white

1 Place the blueberries, Madeira wine, sugar and lime into a small saucepan. Bring to the boil and simmer gently until the blueberries are soft and the liquid has become syrupy. Remove from the heat and allow to cool completely.
2 Place the yogurt in a mixing bowl and stir in the Amaretto and the cooled blueberries.
3 Whisk the egg white into stiff peaks and gently fold into the blueberry and yogurt mixture. Spoon into individual glasses and chill until required.

Gratin of pink grapefruit and orange

SERVES 4
1 SERVING 243 KCAL/0.9G FAT
PREPARATION TIME 20 MINUTES
COOKING TIME 5 MINUTES

You can prepare the fruit in advance and refrigerate. Place under the grill for just 5 minutes and it's ready to serve.

2 large pink grapefruits
4 oranges
4 tbsps Cointreau liqueur
grated fresh nutmeg
4 tsps demerara sugar
basil leaves to decorate

1 Slice both grapefruits in half through the widest part of the fruit.
2 Using a grapefruit knife, carefully remove the grapefruit segments and place in a bowl.
3 Cut away the pith and membrane from the shells and discard. Place the grapefruit shells on a foil-lined baking tray.
4 Using a sharp serrated knife, cut away the skin and pith from the oranges. Segment the fruits into the bowl containing the grapefruit segments by cutting in between the soft membrane and teasing out with the knife.
5 Add the Cointreau and a little nutmeg. Mix well and spoon into the grapefruit shells.
6 Sprinkle with the sugar and place under a hot grill for 4–5 minutes until golden brown. Decorate with basil leaves before serving.

Summer berry smoothie

SERVES 4
1 SERVING 66 KCAL/0.6G FAT
PREPARATION TIME 10 MINUTES

150g (5oz) fresh blueberries
150g (5oz) fresh raspberries
150g (5oz) fresh strawberries, hulled
150ml (¼ pint) ice-cold skimmed milk
150ml (¼ pint) low-fat natural yogurt
1–2 tsps runny honey to taste

1 Rinse the blueberries and raspberries and place in a food processor or liquidiser.
2 Slice the strawberries and place in the food processor with the other fruits.
3 Pour in the milk and yogurt and process for a few seconds until fully combined. Stir in the honey. Pour into glasses and serve.

Summer fruit smoothie

SERVES 2
1 SERVING 105 KCAL/1G FAT
PREPARATION TIME 5 MINUTES

115g (4oz) fresh strawberries, hulled
115g (4oz) fresh raspberries
150ml (¼ pint) low-fat natural yogurt
300ml (½ pint) pineapple juice
runny honey (optional)

1 Wash the strawberries and raspberries well and place in a food processor or liquidiser.
2 Pour in the yogurt and pineapple juice and process for a few seconds until the mixture is thick and creamy. Sweeten with a little runny honey if desired. Pour into tall glasses and serve.

Kiwi and mango salad with lime maple syrup

SERVES 4
1 SERVING 86 KCAL/0.4G FAT
PREPARATION TIME 10 MINUTES

4 ripe kiwi fruits
1 ripe mango
zest and juice of 2 limes
1 tbsp maple syrup
fresh mint to decorate

1 Using a small serrated knife, trim both ends off the kiwi and peel away the skin. Slice the fruits and set aside.
2 Cut away the skin from the mango, using a sharp knife, then slice away the fruit from around the centre stone.
3 Cut the sections of mango into long slices and arrange with the kiwi in alternate layers on a serving plate.
4 Mix the lime zest and juice with the maple syrup and drizzle over the fruits. Decorate with fresh mint and serve immediately.

Raspberry baked meringues

SERVES 8
1 SERVING (1 MERINGUE) 116 KCAL/0.04G FAT
PREPARATION TIME 10 MINUTES
COOKING TIME 3–4 HOURS

Baking meringues with fruit inside adds terrific flavour and texture. They will be crisp on the outside with a chewy concentrated raspberry centre.

4 egg whites
225g (8oz) caster sugar
1 vanilla pod
115g (4oz) fresh raspberries
a little icing sugar to dust

1 Preheat the oven to 140C, 275F, Gas Mark 1.
2 In a very clean mixer bowl whisk the egg whites until stiff. Using a dessertspoon, add the caster sugar a spoonful at a time at 10-second intervals, keeping the mixer on high speed.
3 Place the vanilla pod on a chopping board and splice in half lengthways, using a sharp knife. With the blade of the knife, scrape out the seeds from the vanilla pod and add them to the meringue mixture. Place the pod in a storage container filled with sugar (this will flavour the sugar for use in other meringues or desserts).
4 Lightly grease a baking sheet and cover with parchment paper.
5 Using two large spoons, form the meringues into eight oval shapes by transferring the mixture between the spoons. Place directly on to the parchment paper.

6   Carefully press 4–5 raspberries into the centre of each
    meringue and smooth over with a knife. Bake in the oven for
    3–4 hours until dry on the outside. Turn off the oven and
    leave the meringues in until cool.
7   Serve with a dusting of icing sugar.

Mango and whisky mousse

SERVES 4
1 SERVING 77 KCAL / 0.2G FAT
PREPARATION TIME 10 MINUTES
COOKING TIME 5 MINUTES

1 large fresh ripe mango
2 tbsps whisky
1 × 6g sachet Vege gel
275g (10oz) virtually fat free fromage frais
caster sugar to taste
2 egg whites
fresh fruit or chopped fresh mint to decorate

1   Peel the mango and slice the flesh into a food processor.
    Blend until smooth, then transfer to a saucepan.
2   Add the whisky and sprinkle the Vege gel on top. Heat
    slowly, stirring continuously, until the mixture starts to
    thicken.
3   Pour into a mixing bowl and whisk until smooth. Add the
    fromage frais and a little caster sugar and mix until
    combined.
4   Whisk the egg whites until stiff and fold into the mixture.
    Spoon into individual glasses and decorate with fresh fruit or
    chopped mint.

Fruity coconut milk jelly

SERVES 4
1 SERVING 87 KCAL/3.1G FAT
PREPARATION TIME 5 MINUTES
COOKING TIME 10 MINUTES
SETTING TIME 2 HOURS

1 × 400ml can reduced-fat coconut milk
1 sachet sugar-free raspberry jelly
zest and juice of 1 lime
2 tbsps virtually fat free fromage frais
fresh mint to decorate
virtually fat free fromage frais to serve

1 Pour the coconut milk into a small saucepan and heat until
   boiling.
2 Place the jelly in the mixing bowl. Add the lime zest and
   juice.
3 Pour the hot milk on to the jelly, whisking well with a hand
   whisk. Allow to cool slightly, then whisk in the fromage frais.
   Transfer to a jug and pour into four individual glasses. Place
   in the refrigerator until set.
4 Decorate each glass with fresh mint and a blob of fromage
   frais.

Melon sunrise

SERVES 4
1 SERVING 66 KCAL/0.3G FAT
PREPARATION TIME 15 MINUTES

selection of melon
2 tbsps Campari or Grenadine
sugar to taste
fresh fruit or mint leaves to decorate

1 Peel the melon and remove the seeds. Cut into small cubes
   and arrange in serving glasses.
2 Pour the Campari or Grenadine over the melon, add sugar to
   taste and refrigerate until ready to serve. Decorate with fresh
   fruit or mint before serving.

Mixed grape chill

SERVES 4
1 SERVING 110 KCAL/0.5G FAT
PREPARATION TIME 10 MINUTES

350g (12oz) red and green seedless grapes
150g (5oz) 0% fat Greek yogurt (e.g. Total 0%)
1 tbsp maple syrup

1 Wash the grapes and drain.
2 Cut the grapes in half and place in the bottom of four
   individual glasses.
3 Spoon the yogurt on top and refrigerate until ready to serve.
4 Just before serving drizzle with the maple syrup.

Banana bread pudding

SERVES 8
1 SERVING 117 KCAL/2G FAT
PREPARATION TIME 10 MINUTES
COOKING TIME 30 MINUTES

115g (4oz) wholegrain bread
2 bananas
½ tsp ground mixed spice
2 eggs
450ml (¾ pint) skimmed milk
1 tsp vanilla essence
2 tbsps demerara sugar

1 Preheat the oven to 180C, 350F, Gas Mark 4.
2 Slice the bread into thin slices and arrange in the base of a
   shallow ovenproof dish.
3 Peel and slice the bananas and slot the slices in between the
   bread slices. Sprinkle the mixed spice on top.
4 In a bowl whisk together the eggs and milk. Add the vanilla
   essence and pour the mixture over the bread. Leave to stand
   for 20 minutes to allow the bread to soak up the liquid.
5 Sprinkle the pudding with demerara sugar and bake in the
   oven for 25–30 minutes until golden. Serve hot.

Compote of summer fruits with vanilla yogurt

SERVES 4
1 SERVING 99 KCAL/1.6G FAT
PREPARATION TIME 15 MINUTES
COOKING TIME 10 MINUTES

115g (4oz) fresh raspberries
115g (4oz) fresh strawberries, hulled
115g (4oz) fresh blueberries
115g (4oz) fresh blackberries
1 tbsp flavoured honey (heather or sunflower)
300ml (½ pint) low-fat set yogurt
1 vanilla pod
mint leaves to decorate

1 Place all the fruits in a large colander and rinse well with cold water.
2 Transfer the fruit to a large saucepan so the fruit can spread out. Add the honey and heat gently over a low heat, carefully stirring the fruits to coat with the honey. As soon as the fruits have warmed through, turn off the heat and allow to cool. Spoon into individual glasses.
3 Make the vanilla yogurt by splitting the vanilla pod lengthways. Scrape out the seeds and add to the yogurt. Mix lightly and place in a serving bowl.
4 Decorate with mint leaves and serve with the yogurt.

Wine-poached apricots with raspberries

SERVES 4
1 SERVING 75 KCAL/0.7G FAT
PREPARATION TIME 5 MINUTES
COOKING TIME 10–15 MINUTES

8 fresh apricots
300ml (½ pint) white wine
225g (8oz) low-fat natural yogurt
115g (4oz) raspberries
mint leaves to decorate
icing sugar for dusting

1 Using a small knife, cut the apricots in half, remove the
   centre stones and discard.
2 Place the apricots in a small saucepan and add the white
   wine. Place over a low heat and gently poach for 10–15
   minutes until soft. Allow to cool.
3 Take four dessert glasses and spoon the yogurt in the
   bottom of each glass. Using a slotted spoon, remove the
   apricots from the pan and arrange on top of the yogurt.
4 Scatter with the raspberries and decorate with mint leaves.
   Just before serving, dust with a little icing sugar.

14 Get moving

Making the decision to lose weight is a big step because it involves thought and planning as well as willpower. Having reached this point of commitment, your greatest wish is to see fast results. When you can see and feel the rewards for your efforts – your clothes feel looser and you feel healthier – you know the diet is working and you are encouraged to continue.

So what can you do to maximise your rate of weight loss, speed things along a bit and see even greater benefits? Love it or loathe it, exercise is the key to making this happen. It will make a big difference to your weight-loss progress.

Different kinds of exercise deliver very different results and in this chapter I will explain which type of exercise does what to help give you your desired body shape. Exercise regularly, and you will be staggered at the tremendous benefits you will enjoy in achieving the body you never even dreamed of.

Be a great fat-burner

Any exercise or activity that causes you to breathe more deeply and take in more oxygen is classed as aerobic. Aerobic activities include walking, cycling, running, swimming, rowing, stepping as well as aerobics classes, dancing, salsacise and aqua-aerobics (aerobic exercise in water).

Aerobic exercise does three very important jobs. First, it works the heart and lungs – that's why we become slightly breathless – which is great for our general health and fitness. Second, it causes us to burn fat from our bodies to provide the energy we need to continue the physical activity. Third, and very important for anyone wanting to lose weight, it increases the circulation of oxygen all around the body, particularly to the skin, and this encourages our skin to stay healthy and 'shrink' as we lose weight and become smaller. There really is no downside to exercise. It works miracles when we are trying to shed those pounds or kilos!

When we do aerobic exercise we, in effect, 'turn up the gas' and burn extra calories. It's like converting the engine in your car from a 1.5 litre to a 2.7 litre one. It will use more fuel to run. And that is exactly what happens to the body when we do aerobic exercise. More importantly, exercising aerobically on a regular basis causes the body to become a more efficient fat burner in everyday life – all the time, not just when we are exercising.

Everyone should try to do some kind of aerobic exercise on a regular basis. If you belong to a gym or health club you will have access to a variety of cardiovascular equipment, including the treadmill, stepper, cross trainer, exercise bike, rowing machine, and so on. Group classes include aerobics, step-aerobics, dancing, line dancing, salsacise and, for the very fit, 'Spinning', which is energetic cycling at different gradients in a class situation. All of these are brilliant fat-burners and it is just a matter of preference as to which one you choose. My Gi Jeans Weight-loss Workout DVD has two great aerobic, fat-burning sections – one is a 30-minute traditional aerobic workout and the other is a

20-minute salsacise routine. Either of these will significantly help you slim down. Or, if you're up to it, you can combine both workouts for a mega fat-burning blitz. (There is also a 15-minute Super Toning section.) The great thing about choreographed aerobic routines, as mine are, is that you use almost all the muscles in the body rather than, say, just the legs if you are cycling. You will end up with a great all-round workout that will dramatically improve your figure.

Bear in mind that the most effective aerobic workout for you is the one you enjoy most, because you are likely to go back and do it again and again. That's when you get the real benefits.

Use it or lose it

You've heard the expression 'use it or lose it'. Well, that really is true where our muscles are concerned. If we don't 'challenge' our muscles occasionally by working them, they will become smaller and weaker. As we get older our muscles automatically reduce in size if we don't work them regularly, and over a period of ten years we could reduce our muscle mass by as much as 10lb through wastage while, at the same time, laying down more fat. This would result in a change in our body composition, yet our actual body weight could remain the same. Unlike fat, muscle is energy-hungry tissue, and so a reduction in muscle mass leads to a slowing down of our metabolic rate. This is bad news as it will make us more prone to weight gain unless we eat less food to balance our metabolic needs.

But it doesn't have to be that way. If we challenge our muscles regularly through strength exercises, we can at least sustain them, if not make them stronger and larger. While some men like to build large muscles, women do not have the hormones necessary to create bulging muscles. So don't worry that you'll end up looking like a weight lifter! For this to happen, you would have to work out with massive weights and take supplements. What we are aiming for here is a good muscle tone to give a beautifully toned shape and good body strength to cope with everyday living. The Ultimate Gi Jeans Diet workout in chapter 15 is designed to do just that.

Our muscles are made up of thousands of fibres. If we don't challenge these fibres through regular strength exercise or activities, some of the fibres become redundant and wither away. Conversely, if we use them regularly by working our muscles in exercises where strength is the issue (e.g. using weights at the gym, working out with a toning band, or using our own body weight as resistance), the muscle fibres increase in size to cope with the extra workload. The result: stronger and bigger muscles. This will not only give you a better shape but it will also increase your metabolic rate, as the greater your muscle mass, the higher your metabolic rate.

There is another huge benefit in having strong muscles. When we burn fat during aerobic activity, we burn it in the muscles. That is the only place that fat-burning can take place. So, the bigger and stronger our muscles are, the greater their capacity to burn fat. Isn't that brilliant?

Let's say you have a load of fat on your stomach. You'll need to do lots of ab curls to strengthen the abdominal muscles *underneath* the fat. Then, when you do *aerobic exercise*, your now stronger abdominal muscles will draw on more of the fat that lies on top of the muscles to burn as fuel. Result, fat loss off your stomach! And if you do strength exercises for all the muscles in your body, you will be turning your muscles into fat-burning factories!

So what actually happens in those muscles? The whole aerobic energy system relies on three elements: oxygen (from the air we breathe), carbohydrate (from the food we eat, which is converted to and stored in our muscles as 'glycogen') and, third, fat from around and inside the muscles. When we exercise aerobically, we need fuel and, through a chemical reaction, we manufacture this fuel in our muscles.

Just as we cannot put crude oil into the petrol tanks in our cars – it has to be refined – the oxygen we breathe needs additional components to enable it be converted into the energy we require for exercise, and this conversion takes place in our muscles. Try to imagine your body fat burning in the oxygen flame in your muscles when you exercise. That is why marathon or long-distance runners are so lean. They have burned off most of their body fat!

But if, as soon as you finished your workout, you were to eat a chocolate bar, you would literally be putting back the fat you have just burned off! So after your workout try to eat a low-fat snack that includes some carbohydrate (to replace the carbohydrate burned during exercise). So you could have a chicken salad sandwich or a banana to replenish your energy levels without replacing the fat you have worked so hard to burn away.

Just as we can keep the major muscles of the body strong and firm, we can do the same for the ones in the face. As we get older our facial muscles begin to shrink – the jawline begins to droop and the mouth and lips become thinner. But it doesn't have to be like that. I use a great little gadget called a Facial-Flex, which was created by a surgeon in America to help burns victims regain muscle strength and flexibility in the facial muscles. Not only did it achieve the desired results, but everyone who used it began looking younger, too!

The Facial-Flex works by using a tiny elastic band placed over two ends of a crescent-shaped device which fits into the corners of the mouth. Using the strength of the muscles around your mouth and beyond, you squeeze the two ends together, which stretches the elastic band. As the resistance challenges the facial muscles, the muscles become stronger and bigger, which helps reverse the natural signs of ageing. The elastic bands come in different strengths.

I was sent a Facial-Flex a few years ago to try out and I'm now a dedicated facial workout athlete! I use it every day for a couple of minutes morning and night with the strongest strength band as my facial muscles have become stronger. If you want to find out more, visit the Rosemary Conley website (www.rosemary-conley.co.uk).

Flexibility, posture and balance

Have you ever struggled to zip up the back of your dress, reach up to a high cupboard, or stretch over to retrieve something from the back of your car? These simple everyday tasks can cause back and shoulder problems but, with increased flexibility, we will find these actions easier.

Just as we need our muscles to be strong and fit, we also need our joints to be flexible. Flexibility is incorporated in many forms of exercise. At the end of each exercise class or session we should stretch our muscles to help prevent aching muscles later. This also encourages greater flexibility around our joints and more elasticity in our muscles.

In addition, good posture and balance is important. Losing our sense of balance can have extremely severe consequences for our long-term health.

In recent years the Pilates exercise method has become very popular and there is no doubt that it is excellent for helping people to improve balance, strength and posture. If you want to try it, make sure you find a class with a properly qualified Pilates instructor (see www.pilatesfoundation.com).

Fitness action plan

We can increase our fitness levels by just adding more activity to our daily routine. Try using the stairs more, parking further away, walking more and carrying shopping rather than wheeling it to the car. It all adds up.

We are ten times more likely to continue with a fitness activity if we enjoy it, so find a form of exercise that is fun. Follow these simple guidelines:

- Try to work out at a level that makes you a little breathless for 20–30 minutes on at least five days of the week. If you can't manage such big chunks of time, break it up into smaller 10-minute sections. It still helps.
- Aim to do some toning exercises (chapter 15) two or three times a week to see a real change in your shape.
- Stair climbing is brilliant for toning up your backside. Whenever you have the opportunity to use the stairs, take it.
- Brisk walking is a great form of aerobic exercise and it doesn't cost anything, so walk whenever you can. We burn around 100 calories every time we walk a mile, which is the same as the number of calories burned if we ran it. It's just that running takes less time.
- Think of everyday activities as mini-workouts – gardening, housework, window cleaning, ironing, dog walking,

whatever. They all burn loads more calories than just sitting watching the TV. Get moving and transform yourself – for now and for good!

● Try to do one formal exercise class or work out to a fitness DVD at least once a week. It will help give you a better figure because it works on all the muscle groups. And on those days when you don't feel like working out or going to your class, then that is the time when you really *need* to go!

15 The Ultimate Gi Jeans Diet workout

The prospect of looking good in a pair of jeans provides a great motivation to stick to a diet and exercise programme. In this Ultimate Gi Jeans Diet workout, every exercise has been selected to help you do just that. It is designed to work on all the key areas of the body that make a pair of jeans look right on you. It's not just about hips and thighs – you also need to work at flattening the tummy area so that fastening the zip is smooth and easy, and you definitely don't want any overhang from the waist!

10 easy exercises for the best jeans shape

This programme targets all the key areas in just 10 exercises, five for the hips and thighs and five for the tummy and waist. Do this programme two or three times a week and you will see real results, even more so if you combine it with lots of walking to burn off the excess fat and tone the legs.

How to get the best out of this exercise programme

- Always start with the warm-up exercises. They are designed to loosen your joints and warm your muscles so that they are more pliable and less prone to injury.
- Wear something loose and comfortable and have water available to sip.
- If you are new to exercise, start slowly and gradually build up to the required number of repetitions. As you get stronger you can increase the repetitions.
- Always do the stretches at the end of each section, as these are designed to smooth out the muscles after working them and reduce the risk of injury and sore muscles later.

Hip and thigh workout

- Level 1 uses a chair for support to allow you to do each exercise with control and good technique. Choose a sturdy chair, one with a back high enough for your height.
- Level 2 works exactly the same muscle areas but is much more challenging as it uses a pole (or you can use a broom handle) for support, which means you need to work harder to keep your balance. This demands much more muscle work and hence more calorie burning!
- Start with Level 1 to learn the technique and then progress to Level 2 when you are ready.

Tummy and waist workout

- Select a sturdy chair and position it on a non-slip surface. In some of the exercises, for instance exercises 3 and 5, it's best to place the chair against a wall for safety.
- Do each exercise quite slowly as this makes you work harder.
- Breathe out at the hardest part of the exercise, such as when lifting the head and shoulders in the abdominal exercises.

Warm-up

1 Side bend

Stand tall with feet slightly wider than hip width, tummy pulled in and knees very slightly bent. Now bend from the waist to your left side, reaching your left arm out in the same direction. Try not to lean forward or back and keep your hips still. Come up, and repeat to the other side. Keep changing sides for 12 repetitions (6 each side).

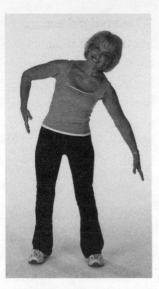

2 Bow and arrow twist

Start in the same position as exercise 1, and bring both arms out in front at shoulder height. Now pull your left elbow back,

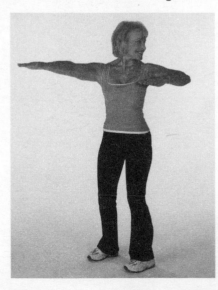

bending the arm and keeping it at shoulder height, with shoulders down and relaxed. Keep watching the elbow so that your head turns as well, and make sure your hips stay facing front, knees slightly bent. Bring the arm back to centre and repeat to the other side. Repeat 12 times (6 each side).

3 Twisted ski swing

Stand with feet parallel and hip distance apart. Bring your arms overhead, keeping your tummy pulled in (a), then bend both knees and swing down with a slight twist in your waist to bring both arms down to your left side (b). Hold your tummy in tight as you lift up again and swing down to the other side. Repeat 12 times (6 each side).

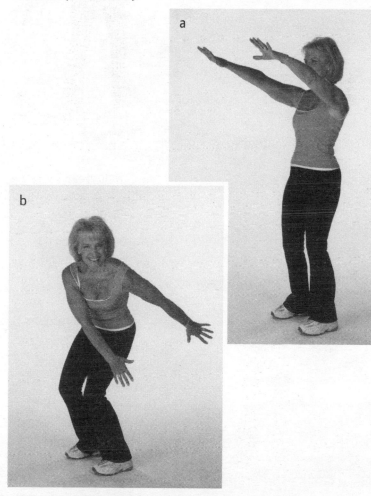

4 Squat with arm reach

Still with feet parallel and hip distance apart, pull your tummy in and bend both knees, pressing your hips back and reaching your arms forward. Don't let your hips go lower than your knees, and make sure your knees are over your ankles. Come up again without locking the knees, and repeat 12 times.

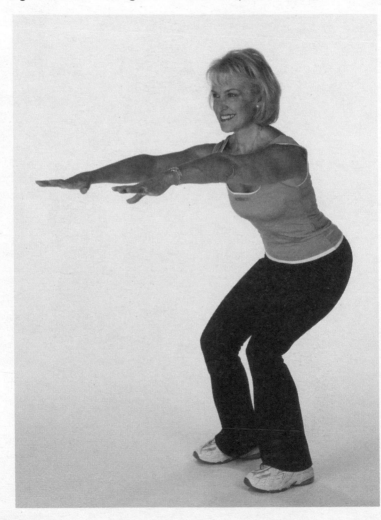

5 Rocking horse

Take one step forward with your right foot and lift your left leg behind, keeping it straight and raising arms in front (a). Now transfer your weight on to your left leg and bring the right leg in to meet it (b). Do 10 repetitions, then repeat with the other leg leading.

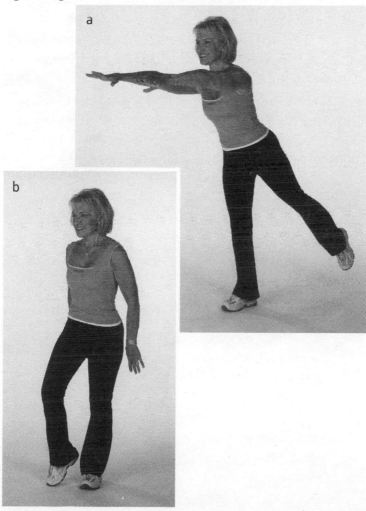

Hip and thigh workout

Level 1

1 Total hip and thigh toner

Stand with feet parallel and just wider than your hips, and hold on to the back of the chair for support. Pull your tummy in tight and keep your back straight as you bend from the knees, pushing your hips back (a). Come up again without locking your knees at the top and, at the same time, bring one leg out to the side with foot turned down slightly and hips still facing forward (b). Bend your knees again and then lift the other leg. Do 12 repetitions, rest, and then do another 12.

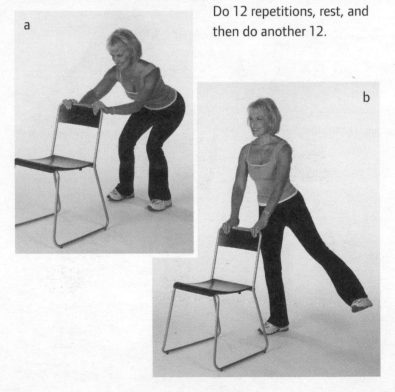

2 Outer thigh toner

Hold the chair with your right hand and place your left hand on your left hip. Stand tall in a good posture with tummy in and knees slightly bent. Now lift your left leg out to the side, with foot turned down slightly. Keep your hips facing forward and your trunk upright. Do 12 repetitions, then turn around to repeat with the other leg. Build up to another 12 repetitions on each leg.

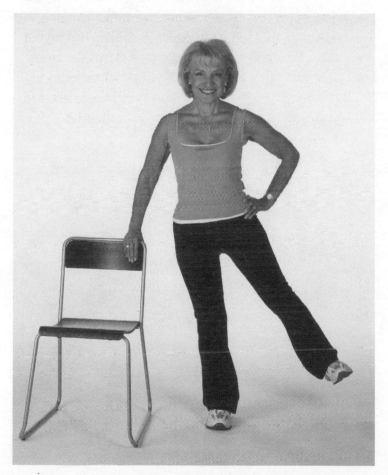

3 Inner thigh toner

Hold the chair with your right hand. Transfer your weight on to your left leg and lift your right foot off the floor and across your left leg, leading with the heel (a). Keep the knee of the standing leg slightly bent and your body upright, with hips facing forward. Lift the leg across slowly in 3 small movements, gradually taking the leg higher on each lift (b). Repeat 6 times, then turn round and repeat with the other leg.

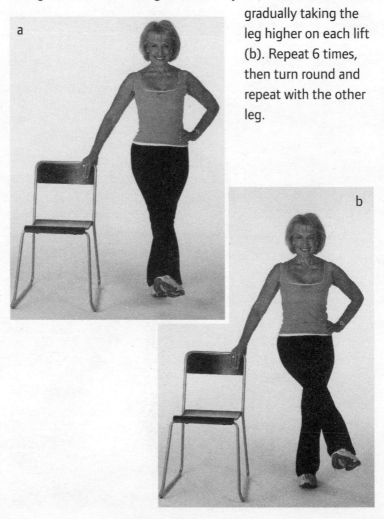

4 Bottom lifter

Stand a short distance behind the chair. Hold on to the back
and lean forward slightly with tummy pulled in tight. Lift your
left leg back and up, keeping your hips facing forward. Bring
the leg down again and bend your knees slightly before taking
your right leg back, up and down again. Keep changing legs in
a smooth and rhythmical way for 12 repetitions. Rest, and then
do another set of 12.

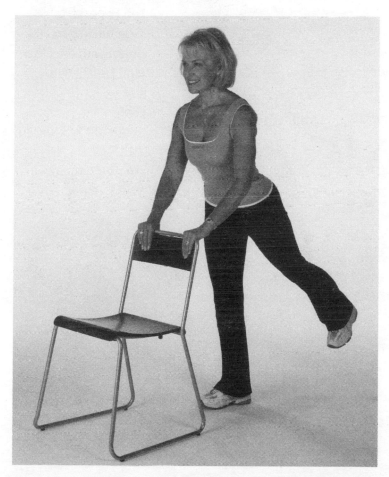

5 Thigh shaper lunge

Hold the chair with your right hand. Take one large step forward with your right foot and raise the heel of your back foot. Keep your trunk upright, with tummy in and shoulders back and down (a). Now bend both knees to 90 degrees, making sure the front knee is in line with the ankle not the toes (b). Straighten the legs, with your weight distributed equally between both legs, and keep bending and straightening for 12 slow repetitions. Turn round to change legs and repeat.

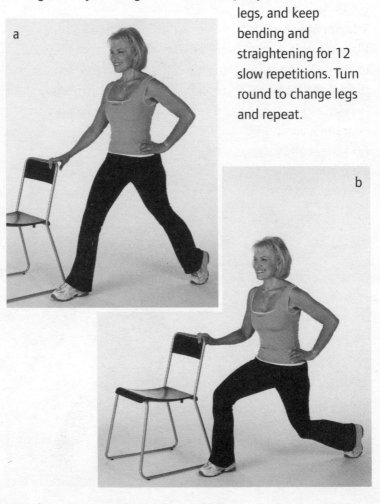

Level 2

Placing the pole across your shoulders gives a good postural alignment and reminds you to use your tummy muscles to keep your balance. This level is a lot harder than Level 1 but really effective if you can master it. Try doing these exercises in front of a mirror to check that you are keeping the pole straight.

1 Inner thigh slide

Place the pole across your shoulders and stand with feet together. Take a large step out to the side with your left leg and then slide your right leg along the floor to meet the left foot. Repeat to the other side, keeping your knees slightly bent and your trunk upright. Do 12 repetitions, alternating sides, then rest and do another set.

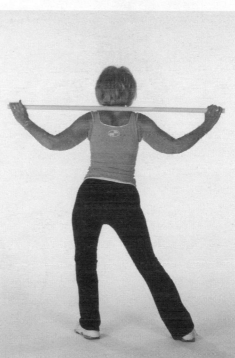

2 Total hip and thigh toner

Place the pole across your shoulders and stand with feet parallel and just wider than your hips. Pull your tummy in, bend your knees in line with your ankles and press your hips back into a squat position (a). Make sure your hips do not go lower than the knees. As you lift again, bring your left leg out to the side, with toes down slightly (b). Bend again and then lift, this time taking the right leg out to the side. Go slowly and you will really feel the work in the thighs! Do 12 repetitions to alternate sides (6 each side), then rest and repeat.

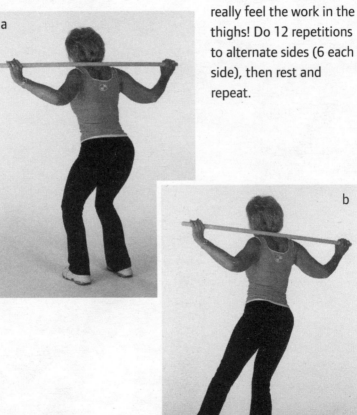

a

b

3 Outer thigh shaper

Stand with the pole across your shoulders and feet parallel.
Bend your knees slightly and then come up again, bringing one
leg up and out to the side. Keep your trunk upright and your
tummy in tight to help you balance. Bring the leg in again,
bending the knees before taking it up to the same side. Repeat
12 times, then change legs and repeat. Rest, and do another
set on each leg.

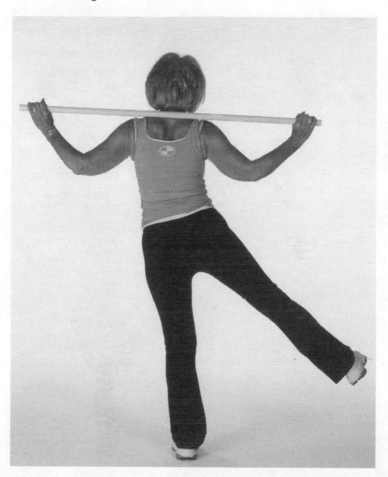

4 Bottom lifter

Stand with feet parallel and hip distance apart. Hold the pole in both hands and rest it on your thighs (a). Pull your tummy in tight and bend your knees slightly. Now lift the pole straight out in front to shoulder height and, at the same time, raise one leg behind (b). Keep your tummy in and lean forward to help you balance. Bring the leg down, bending your knees, before lifting the other leg. Do 12 repetitions with alternate legs (6 each leg), then rest and repeat.

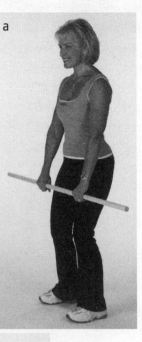

a

b

5 Lunge repeater

Place the pole a little distance in front of you for support and stand tall with feet parallel. Take a large step forward with one leg and raise the heel of the back foot (a). Now bend both knees to 90 degrees, with the front knee over the ankle (b) and straighten again. Make sure your trunk remains upright and your tummy pulled in tight.

Keep bending and straightening for 6 repetitions, then change legs and repeat. Rest and then build up to another set on each leg.

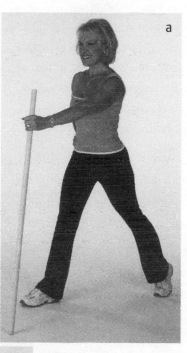

Hip and thigh stretches

1 Hip stretch

Hold the back of the chair with your right hand. Now slide your left leg back as far as you can, keeping your body upright, and slowly bend both knees, making sure the front knee stays over the ankle. Push the left hip forward to feel a stretch at the front of the left hip. Hold for 10 seconds, then release. Change legs and repeat.

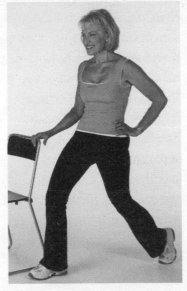

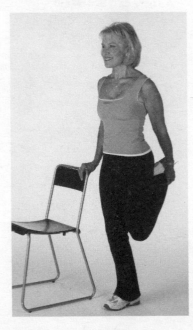

2 Front thigh stretch

Hold the back of the chair with your right hand. Lift your left leg and hold around the ankle with your left hand. Keep your knees together, with back straight, tummy in and standing leg slightly bent. Press the left hip forward for a more effective stretch. Hold for 10 seconds, then release. Change legs and repeat.

3 Back thigh stretch

Still holding the back of the chair, place your left foot one step in front of the right, with both feet pointing forward. Now bend your back knee, keeping the front leg straight, thighs together, and place your left hand on the left thigh for support. Bring your hips up slightly to feel a strong stretch at the back of the left thigh. Hold for 10 seconds, then release. Change sides and repeat.

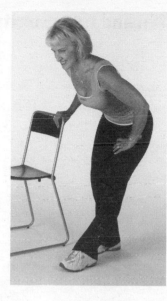

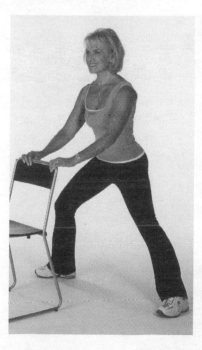

4 Inner thigh stretch

Hold the back of the chair with both hands and bend your right knee. Now slide your left leg further to the left without transferring your weight, keeping the leg straight and the foot pointing forward, until you feel a stretch in the left inner thigh. Keep your trunk upright and check that your right knee is bent over the ankle and not the toes. Hold for 10 seconds, then release. Change sides and repeat.

Tummy and waist workout

1 Curl up

Lie on your back with your hands behind your head and your lower legs on the chair seat (a). Breathe in and, as you breathe out, pull your tummy in tight and slowly lift your head and shoulders off the floor (b). Lower again slowly, breathing in at the same time. Repeat 8 times, then rest and repeat.

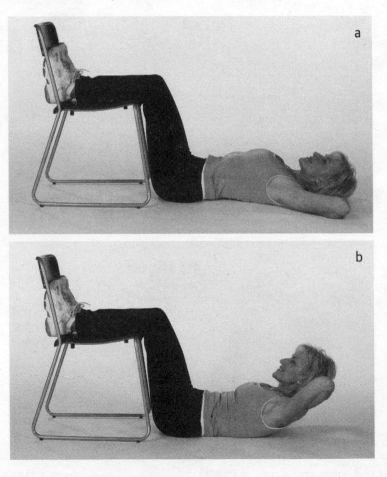

a

b

2 Waist reach

In same starting position as exercise 1, breathe in and, as you breathe out, pull your tummy in and lift your head and shoulders off the floor, reaching your left hand in the direction of the left front chair leg. Feel your spine curve round to the left and the waist muscles on your left side tighten. Breathe in as you slowly lower again, and then repeat to the other side. Keep changing sides for 12 repetitions (6 each side).

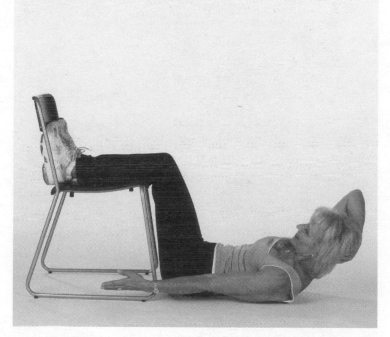

3 Back strengthener and waist firmer

Lie on your front with arms by your sides and head face down on the floor. Now lift your head and chest just off the floor, keeping your head facing down, and slide your left hand down your left side to curve your spine slightly. Return to the centre and release. Lift again and curve to the other side. Keep changing sides for 12 repetitions (6 each side).

N.B. Don't do this exercise if you have a bad back or have had back problems in the last six months.

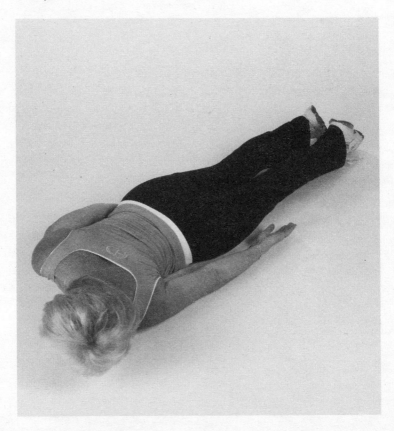

4 Waist shaper

Lie on your back with both legs over the chair seat, your right hand behind your head and your left arm out to the side in line with your shoulder (a). Breathe in and, as you breathe out, pull your tummy in tight and lift your head and shoulders off the floor, twisting slightly in the waist and taking your right shoulder in the direction of the left leg (b). Lower again under control, and do 8 repetitions to the same side. Repeat on the other side.

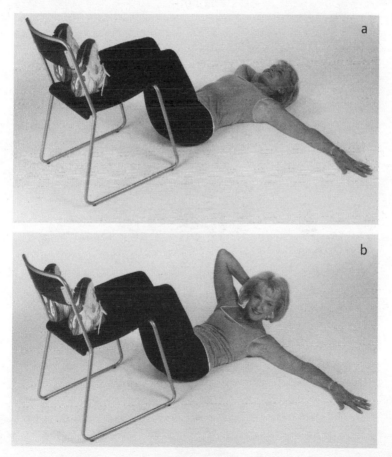

5 Tummy crunch

Begin with both legs on the chair seat, ankles crossed, knees bent and both hands behind your head (a). Breathe in and, as you breathe out, curl your head and shoulders off the floor and, at the same time, lift your legs off the chair seat (b). Slowly lower again, allowing your heels to touch the chair seat as a release. Repeat 8 times, then rest and repeat.

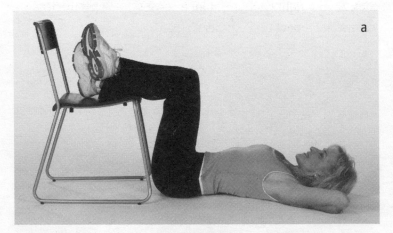

a

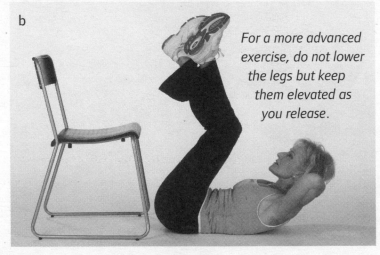

b

For a more advanced exercise, do not lower the legs but keep them elevated as you release.

Tummy and waist stretches

1 Lying waist stretch

Lie on your back with knees bent and feet and knees together.
Place your arms out in a 'T' shape at shoulder height, with
palms down. Pull your tummy in to support your back, and roll
your knees over to the left. At the same time, turn your head to
look at your right hand. Hold for 8 seconds, then return to
centre and repeat to the other side.

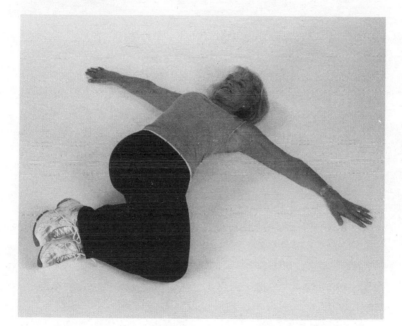

2 Tummy stretch

Lie on your front with elbows bent in line with your shoulders. Now prop up on your elbows, keeping your hips and elbows in contact with the floor. Breathe in and, as you breathe out, draw your chin up slightly to feel a stretch down the front of your trunk. Hold for 8 seconds, then release.

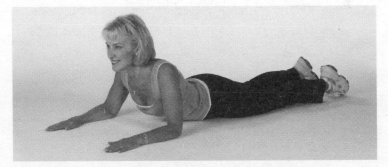

3 Seated waist stretch

Sit upright with legs crossed (or sit in a chair if you prefer). Place your left hand on the floor in line with the hip. Reach your right arm up and bend to your left side, keeping both hips firmly on the floor and without leaning forward or back. Keep reaching the right arm high to feel a strong stretch in the waist on the right side. Hold for 8 seconds, then release. Repeat on the right side.

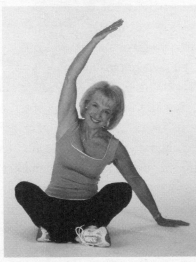

16 Eat and stay slim

How do you find the winning formula to keep your weight down one you have successfully lost it? That is the challenge. If you follow these simple rules you should be able to continue to maintain your new and healthier body in the long term.

Losing weight is relatively straightforward with my Ultimate Gi Jeans Diet because you have a specific calorie allowance to try to stick to and a goal to aim for. If you have a good week you can lose a significant amount of weight. If you have an OK week, you may lose just a little weight or stay the same. If you have a bad week, you probably gain weight. You know how it works.

But weight maintenance is different, isn't it? Or so you might think. Initially, when we reach our goal weight, we are so thrilled to be at the end of our strict eating programme that has inevitably restricted our food choices. Years and years ago when I reached my own goal weight, after losing almost 2½st, I can remember visiting the supermarket and looking adoringly at all the foods I had forgone over the previous months. 'Shall I have a cream cake to celebrate? A chocolate bar, maybe? Or just a big bag of crisps? Perhaps all of them! After all, I'm at my ideal weight now,' I tried to convince myself.

Somehow, all those years ago, I was completely missing the point. I was thinking in a similar way to the person who finds themselves in debt, goes on an economy drive to pay off the debt and then, once the money is repaid, embarks on a spending spree! It's madness. If we carry on like this, whether it's eating those foods that made us overweight in the first place, or continuing our overspending habits, we will find ourselves right back where we started – overweight or overdrawn again.

The key to avoiding this sad and disappointing state of affairs is to change your LIFESTYLE, not just your diet or your shopping trips. You have to learn some new habits and incorporate them into your daily life – for good!

My four simple rules for weight loss are:

1 Eat low-fat foods.
2 Choose foods with a low Gi rating.
3 Watch the calories.
4 Be as active as possible!

These are the basic rules for anyone who wants to *lose* weight. And they are just as relevant for anyone wanting to *maintain* their weight. So let's look at them more closely.

1 Eat low-fat foods

The good news is that if you have been following a low-fat diet for any length of time your taste buds will have changed. The taste of fatty or oily foods becomes unpalatable, so sticking with low-fat eating is not a hardship; it's a pleasure. However, in just the same way that we can re-educate our taste buds away from fatty foods, we can reverse that trend and revert to our old habits if we allow ourselves to slip backwards.

I remember starting to have butter on my bread roll if I dined out. It didn't take long before I was looking forward to having butter on other foods, too. Realising the slippery slope I was on, I took the opportunity of stopping the habit for Lent that year and I have not gone back to eating butter on my bread again. It was a real warning lesson to me. I hadn't realised how easily I could slip back and, as I so wanted to stay slim, I vowed never to stray again and to make low-fat eating a lifestyle pattern in the long term. Now, it is no effort at all to eat low fat as a matter of course and, consequently, I maintain my weight relatively easily.

So it's important to continue with the habit of cooking and serving food without added fat. You just don't need it. Aim to avoid high-fat foods such as chocolate, crisps and nuts except as occasional treats. If you start eating them every day, you are heading right back into your large clothes again.

Use low-fat dressings on salads and avoid oil, including olive oil, if you can. Remember, oil is 100 per cent fat. If you eat foods with a maximum of five per cent fat as a matter of habit, without having to be an absolute slave to it, you'll find weight mainte-nance easier than you think. One exception to this rule is of course your weekly portion of oily fish, which is important for good health.

2 Choose foods with a low Gi rating

As I have said earlier in this book, you do not have to become a Gi slave to stay healthy. If you have followed the diet in this book you will have automatically incorporated more low-Gi foods into your everyday eating. Just try to continue eating wholegrain or multigrain bread when you have the opportunity. Choose bas-mati rice in preference to other varieties. Include more pasta-based meals in your eating plan. Try to eat oat-based cereals or other low-Gi options such as Special K or Shredded Wheat more often. Choose new or sweet potatoes in place of regular, old ones as a general rule, but that doesn't mean that you can never have an 'old' jacket potato. Of course you can and it is still healthy and nutritious.

By the time you reach this maintenance plan you will have learned a lot about low-Gi eating. Some of you will have grown to love it, while others may find it omits some of their favourite foods. That's OK. Just try to incorporate low-Gi options when you can and your weight maintenance and your overall health will benefit.

3 Watch the calories

Once you've reached your goal, the ideal scenario is to wean yourself away from counting every single calorie. Along your journey to achieve a slim and healthy body, hopefully you will have learned a great deal about portion sizes and developed a general understanding of calorie values. You will also have learned about calorie short-cuts too, such as mashing potatoes with yogurt rather than butter, stir-frying in a non-stick wok without oil, and dry-roasting potatoes. You shouldn't need to count calories ever again if you don't slip back into your old high-fat, high-calorie habits.

If you are trying to maintain your weight but find the pounds or kilos creeping back on and you know you are not overindulging in lots of high-fat treats or overdoing the alcohol, the chances are that your portion sizes have crept up. Just as the stomach shrinks quite quickly as you eat less when trying to lose weight, it can expand again if you consistently give it more and more at each meal time. It's a habit that is easier to break than to make, so you need to remind yourself how great it is to be slim and how life was not so enjoyable when you were fatter.

For some people, though, calorie counting is no effort and it gives them a sense of security. 'If I keep to my calories I know I can't gain weight again,' some dieters say, and maybe in the early stages of maintenance this is a safe option while they come to terms with eating a little more. The ideal is to gradually increase your calories over a period of weeks, allowing you and your body to re-adjust to having more food.

Here are some guidelines on how to increase your calories to keep your weight constant. If you find that your weight goes up with these extra calories, rather than cutting down again, try to step up your activity levels so that you *burn more* calories.

INCREASING THE DAILY CALORIES ON YOUR MAINTENANCE PLAN

Likely daily calories at end of weight-loss plan	= 1400
Maintenance Week 1	
+ 200 calories extra per day	= 1600
Maintenance Week 2	
+ 50 calories extra per day	= 1650
Maintenance Week 3	
+ 50 calories extra per day	= 1700
Maintenance Week 4	
+ 50 calories extra per day	= 1750
Maintenance Week 5	
+ 50 calories extra per day	= 1800

4 Be as active as possible!

Exercise is the very best aid to weight maintenance as it does much more than just burn calories. It strengthens the muscles, which increases the metabolic rate, it helps you to burn fat more easily when you do aerobic activity, and it also helps to tone the skin. It is the best long-term investment for your health, figure and fitness. Without doubt, it will prove a huge aid in helping you to maintain your new slim body.

While you were losing your excess weight, almost certainly you will have increased your activity levels. Whether through formal exercise at a class or using one of my fitness DVDs, rediscovering a sport from your childhood, taking up ballroom dancing, gardening more or walking the dog further, hopefully, you have enjoyed it. When you reach your goal weight, try very hard to maintain this higher level of activity.

Not only will you find you have boundless energy as a result of losing your unwanted weight but you will have become SO much fitter and healthier. You will be sleeping better and your body shape will be transformed!

Surely you don't want to lose that feeling, so keep up your exercise! There's no need to become obsessive about it. Just try to do two or three proper workouts a week – a couple of classes and a fitness video or a game of sport will be sufficient – and then be more active generally in your everyday life. Use the stairs more frequently. Try to walk more and drive less.

One dieter wrote to me enthusing about her success on my Gi Jeans Diet. She started walking her dog more frequently, for increased distances, and at a brisker pace. Not only did it help her to lose weight faster, her dog slimmed down too, much to the delight of the vet!

To sum up…

Here are my golden rules for weight maintenance:

- Continue to eat foods low in fat whenever possible and eat three meals a day. Try to limit Power Snacks to just one between each meal.
- Make low-fat cooking part of your lifestyle. It will keep you leaner and healthier.
- Keep any high-fat foods as occasional treats rather than regular indulgences.
- Choose foods which are low Gi whenever possible. They will keep you feeling satisfied for longer and will contribute to your good health.
- Increase your daily calories gradually (see page 311 for guidance). These calories can be taken as slightly larger portions or as extra pieces of fruit or an extra drink.
- Watch your portion sizes. This is likely to be the one area where you may consume extra calories without realising it.
- Stay active! Maintain the same levels of exercise and activity that you achieved in your weight-loss campaign. This will significantly help you to maintain your new level of fitness, stay in good shape and keep your weight down.
- Weigh yourself weekly on the same scales and under the same conditions – same time of day, same clothing, etc. Record your progress.
- Measure yourself at least monthly to check your inches or centimetres and write them down. Sometimes you may gain weight but your inches or centimetres stay the same, so there may be no need to worry. It could just be a fluid level imbalance.

- Keep a bag containing goods, such as tins of food, of the equivalent amount of your total weight loss. It will be a tremendous encouragement and constant reminder of your achievement. If you gain some weight, remove an equal amount of weight from the bag. It will help you to recognise how much you have still achieved and will hopefully stop you from becoming despondent. As you lose the weight again, place the goods back in the bag.
- And finally, if you do find a few pounds creeping back on, don't panic and don't dwell on it. Relax and just cut back on your food quantities, treats and alcohol for a few days and you'll shift the excess weight.

The most successful long-term dieter is the one who has changed their lifestyle to incorporate these simple guidelines. It needn't be difficult but it is crucial that you enjoy your new, slimmer, fitter body to the full. Feeling healthier, buying new clothes that you couldn't have worn before, accepting compliments and enjoying feeling like a 'normal' person is truly wonderful. As one of my successful slimmers said: 'Now people talk TO me instead of about me.' That is utterly priceless, so enjoy the new you!

17 Dining out

You can still dine out when you are on a weight-reducing diet. You just need to choose wisely and compensate for any indulgence with some extra exercise the next day. Here are some simple tips to help you enjoy such an occasion while keeping weight gain to a minimum. Check out also my guidelines for different types of cuisine. These will help steer you towards the right choices.

Ten tips for dining out

1 Plan ahead for the day of your meal out. Make an effort to reduce your calorie intake for the rest of your meals and save up your treat and alcohol allowance.

2 Before your meal, try sipping low-calorie drinks such as water or slimline mixers to help fill you up.

3 Avoid the bread roll if you can. It probably takes up around 130 calories – and that will double if you add butter!

4 Ideally, select a fruit-based starter, such as melon, sorbet, or alternatively a light soup. Any of these options will give you few calories but help fill you up!

5 Opt for dishes that are grilled, steamed or baked and avoid anything fried, deep-fried or sautéed. If you are not sure how something is cooked or what ingredients it contains, ask.

6 Ask for your vegetables to be served without butter, and salad without dressing, and eat plenty of them to fill you up.

7 If you want a dessert, use your treat calories. If you're feeling saintly, choose sorbets, yogurt or fresh fruit salad.

8 Enjoy a glass or two of wine but drink plenty of water in between sips.

9 Don't forget that alcohol calories can soon add up. So, save up your alcohol allowance for a few days beforehand and keep a check on what you are drinking.

10 Don't worry if you have overindulged a little – it's not the end of the world. Just cut back on a few calories the next day and be more physically active. In a couple of days your body will have lost any weight you might have gained from that one meal. It is only when you dine out and overindulge regularly that you will seriously affect your progress.

Food on the go

Burgers

- The smaller and plainer the burger, the better.
- Avoid cheese, sauces and mayonnaise.
- Don't be tempted by extras such as fries.
- Drinks – choose a low-calorie soft drink, mineral water, tea or coffee and avoid milkshakes.

Fish and chips

- Order a small fish and remove the batter before you eat it.
- Share chips – order the smallest portion and share them with a friend.
- If you're eating your fish meal at home, cook your own low-fat oven chips.
- Have a pot of mushy peas or baked beans – they are good low-fat, low-Gi choices.

Sandwiches

- Look for prepacked low-fat sandwiches, ideally made with wholegrain bread for a low-Gi option.
- Avoid fillings that include mayonnaise and cheese.
- If the sandwiches are made to order ask for 'no butter'.
- Choose low-fat fillings such as chicken, tuna or cottage cheese with lots of salad but pass on the mayonnaise.

Fried chicken

- Choose chicken wings.
- Remove the breadcrumbs, batter and skin before eating to reduce the fat and calorie content.
- Steer clear of bargain buckets!

CAUTION!

- 2 pieces of Kentucky Fried Chicken with regular chips contain around 750 calories and 40g fat!

Pub food

Starters

- Choose healthier options such as melon, stock-based soups, grapefruit cocktail, and smoked salmon.
- Avoid prawn cocktail, avocado, and pâté, which are high in fat and calories.

Main courses

- Choose grilled, poached or chargrilled dishes.
- Trim off any excess fat from meat and remove the skin from chicken.
- Avoid rich sauces and ask for all sauces to be served separately.
- Choose new potatoes rather than chips or sautéed potatoes for a low-fat, low-Gi option.
- Ask for vegetables to be served without butter and salad without dressing or for the dressing to be served separately.

Desserts

- Avoid pies or anything baked in pastry as they are high in fat and calories.
- Beware of traditional puddings such as apple pie – it may be full of apples but it's also full of calories.
- Choose fresh fruit, ice cream, sorbet, or crème caramel.

CAUTION!

- A portion of fried scampi contains around 560 calories and 27g fat!

Italian

Starters

- Choose melon with Parma ham, or minestrone soup.
- Avoid garlic bread – ask for plain bread or grissini (bread sticks) instead.

Main courses

- Avoid pasta with creamy or butter-based sauces such as carbonara and *alfredo*.
- Choose pasta with tomato-based sauces such as arrabbiata, Napoletana, marinara, and pomodori.
- Steer clear of cannelloni and lasagne – they are loaded with fat and calories.
- Avoid *parmigiana* dishes – they are floured, fried and baked with cheese.
- Choose grilled calf's liver and grilled fish for healthy options.
- Go easy on dishes with pesto – they contain olive oil.
- Choose thin-crust pizzas rather than deep-pan ones and ask for less cheese on top.

- Go for healthy pizza toppings such as chicken, tuna and vegetables – but resist the olive oil.
- Avoid pizza toppings such as pepperoni, salami, anchovies and olives – they will add extra fat and calories.

Side dishes
- Choose salads but ask for salad dressings to be served separately.

Desserts
- Choose fresh fruit salads, sorbet or *granita di limone* (lemon water ice).
- Avoid traditional high-fat desserts such as zabaglione and tiramisu.
- Go easy on ice cream – some varieties are high in fat.

CAUTION!
- An average portion of lasagne contains 650 calories and 44g fat!
- Parmesan cheese contains 33 per cent fat!

Greek

Starters
- Choose zatziki (made from yogurt), pitta bread, *avgolemono* (chicken and lemon soup) and grilled sardines.
- Avoid taramasalata – it contains 223 calories and 23g fat per average portion!

Main courses

- Choose baked fish with tomato and garlic, dolmades (stuffed vine leaves), stifado (beef stew) and kleftiko (roast lamb).
- Opt for chicken and pepper kebabs and souvlaki (pork kebabs) rather than the higher-fat lamb kebabs (doner or kofta).
- Avoid high-fat dishes such as fried fish, moussaka and *spanakopita* (spinach pie with feta cheese).

Side dishes

- Avoid Greek salad (it contains feta cheese, olives and olive oil) and choose a plain salad instead.
- Be wary of aubergine dishes – if they're cooked in olive oil they will have soaked up lots of fat.

Desserts

- Avoid pastries such as *baklava* (layered filo pastry with honey and nuts).
- Choose fresh figs, fresh fruit or sorbet.

CAUTION!

- An average portion of traditional moussaka contains around 700 calories and 41g fat!

French

Starters

- Choose consommé (clear soup), crudités, and open shell mussels.
- Avoid high-fat dishes such as French onion soup, escargots (snails), pâté, and garlic mushrooms.

Main courses

- Choose meat or fish dishes that are grilled or baked, such as plain steak or grilled sole, or dishes cooked in wine, such as steak with red wine, chicken chasseur, and braised beef casserole.
- Steer clear of dishes with rich, heavy sauces, such as beef bourguignon, cassoulet, duck à l'orange, and steak with béarnaise sauce.
- Choose meat or fish served *en papillote* – wrapped in paper and baked in the oven using only a little fat or oil.
- Avoid anything *en croute* – which means it comes in pastry.

Side dishes

- Resist the *pommes frites* (French fries) if you can and opt for new potatoes instead.
- Choose salad or steamed vegetables.
- Avoid goat's cheese salad.

Desserts

- Choose fresh fruit salad, sorbet, crème caramel, meringue with fresh fruit – but no added cream!
- Avoid gateaux, cakes, pastries and crème brûlée.
- Resist the cheese board, if you can, or have just a small piece of cheese with celery or grapes.

CAUTION!

- An average portion of duck à l'orange with its skin on contains 856 calories and 69g fat!
- Brie is 27 per cent fat!

Spanish

Starters

- Choose gazpacho, marinated calamari, serrano ham (a great alternative to chorizo), and green beans with ham.
- Avoid salted almonds, deep-fried calamari, battered shrimps, and chorizo sausages.
- Go easy on the tapas – commonly nibbled with a glass of wine, they'll pile on the pounds before you've even started your main course!

Main courses

- Steer clear of dishes that are *frito* (fried) or *a la plancha* (pan fried).
- Avoid *escabèches* (a spicy cold dish of fish or poultry, fried and then marinated) and *empanadas* (flaky pastry filled with meat, fish or chicken and vegetables).
- Choose chicken *sofrito* (stir-fried chicken), paella, stuffed peppers with rice, and *olla podrida* (special soup with meat, poultry, rice and lentils), *Galician cocido* (meat stew with potatoes, parsnips, chickpeas and beans) for good low-fat, low-Gi options.
- Go easy on Spanish omelette and *piperade* (fried dish with eggs, peppers, onion, garlic, ham and herbs) as these may be cooked in olive oil.

Side dishes

- Choose *escalibada* (grilled or barbecued vegetables) or fresh salad.
- Avoid vegetables cooked or drizzled in olive oil.

Desserts
- Choose fresh fruit salad and ice-cream.
- Avoid sweet pastries and *churros* (hot fritters).

> **CAUTION!**
> - A starter portion of fried calamari contains 234 calories and 12g fat!

Indian

Starters
- Avoid anything deep-fried such as onion bhajis, pakoras and samosas.
- Ask for poppadums to be grilled rather than fried.
- Choose chicken or prawn tandoori/tikka or soups.

Main courses
- Share a main course with a friend – Indian portions tend to be generous.
- Choose tandoori or tikka dishes (without additional sauces) as these are usually grilled or barbecued in a clay oven rather than fried.
- Opt for chicken and prawn dishes – they are lower in fat than lamb.
- Choose tomato-based dishes such as jalfrezi and rogan josh rather than cream-based ones.
- Avoid dishes made with cream, coconut or almonds, such as korma, masala or pasanda, and dishes that involve lots of fried ingredients, such as such as *dupiaza*.

Side dishes and sundries

- Choose chapati or roti bread rather than naan or paratha.
- Opt for boiled or steamed basmati rice rather than fried.
- Choose dahl (made with lentils) in preference to panir dishes (made with Indian cheese) for a good low-fat, low-Gi option.
- Go for raita (cucumber and yogurt), mango chutney, lime pickle, and onion salad instead of rich sauces to enhance dishes.

Desserts

- Choose fresh fruit salad, lychees or mangoes.
- Avoid kulfi (Indian ice cream) – it's surprisingly high in fat and calories.

CAUTION!

- An average main course portion of chicken tikka masala contains around 680 calories and 41g fat. Do without the masala sauce and you'll save 258 calories and 26g fat!
- Most Indian dishes are cooked using ghee (clarified butter), which is a whopping 99.8 per cent fat!

Chinese

Starters

- Choose chicken and sweetcorn soup or dim sum (if steamed).
- Avoid deep-fried dishes such as spring rolls, seaweed, sesame prawns on toast and fried dim sum.
- Go easy on the prawn crackers – they contain around 10 calories each and are extremely moreish!

Main courses

- Choose dishes with sauces such as black bean, oyster or hoisin as these tend to be lower in fat and calories than deep-fried dishes such as crispy Peking duck or crispy lamb.
- Avoid sweet and sour dishes. The meat is often deep-fried and the sauces are high in sugar.
- Opt for steamed or stir-fried dishes – they'll fill you up but with less fat.
- Avoid dishes with cashew nuts – they contain more than 50 per cent fat!

Side dishes and sundries

- Choose stir-fried bamboo shoots, water chestnuts or steamed spring greens instead of deep-fried vegetable dishes for great low-fat, low-Gi options.
- Opt for low-fat, low-Gi options such as boiled or steamed noodles instead of egg-fried rice.
- Steer clear of Singapore fried noodles – they contain a whopping 529 calories and 19.5g fat per average portion.

Desserts

- Avoid deep-fried desserts, such as banana fritters.
- Choose fresh fruit, lychees or sorbet.

CAUTION!

- An average main course portion of sweet and sour pork contains around 705 calories and 42g fat!

Thai

Starters
- Choose a soup such as *tom yum* (hot and sour prawn soup with lemongrass) or chicken and sweetcorn or crabmeat and sweetcorn soup.
- Avoid deep-fried dishes such as spring rolls, prawns on toast, sweetcorn cakes, crispy aromatic duck or seaweed, and pan-fried dumplings.

Main courses
- Avoid dishes such as Thai red or green curry as they contain coconut milk, which has a high fat content.
- Ask for a dish that does not contain coconut or peanut-based sauces.
- Choose chicken, beef and prawn stir-fries or noodle dishes but avoid dishes containing cashew nuts.
- Avoid sweet and sour dishes as these are often fried and the sauce is high in sugar.

Side dishes
- Choose stir-fried mixed vegetables or pak choi.
- Choose steamed rice instead of fried rice.

Desserts
- Choose fresh fruit, mangoes or lychees.
- Avoid deep-fried dishes such as apple or banana fritters.

> **CAUTION!**
> - A traditional Thai green curry contains around 33g fat!

Mexican

Starters
- Choose *ceviche* (raw fish marinated in lime juice).
- Avoid quesadilla (tortilla bread covered in cheese, meat, and spring onions).

Main courses
- Opt for barbecued or grilled meats.
- Choose fajitas (soft tortilla with chicken, peppers and onion) but don't add guacamole or sour cream.
- Choose *burritos* (oven-baked tortilla) without the cheese.
- Avoid *chimichangas* (deep-fried stuffed tortilla) and *enchiladas* (stuffed tortilla covered in cheese).

Side dishes
- Choose salsa to accompany dishes.
- Avoid sour cream, guacamole and refried beans – all high in fat and calories.

CAUTION!
- A 350g portion of chicken quesadilla contains around 750 calories and 30g fat!

18 Your questions answered

Each week I receive hundreds of letters from readers or slimmers who are about to embark on a weight-loss diet or who are already on their way and I try to answer as many as possible. Here's a selection of typical ones.

Q Can I eat ordinary brown rice instead of basmati rice on your Gi Jeans Diet?

A Basmati rice is particularly tasty and aromatic and has a low-Gi rating. It is lower in calories than white long-grain rice, although ordinary brown rice has a similar Gi value to basmati rice. Brown rice is higher in fibre than white rice, and this in itself has health benefits. Basmati rice – brown or white – contains more amylose, a starch that slows the rate of digestion, and so it's the best option for weight loss.

Q I am a vegetarian and want to lose weight. Can I follow your diet?

A Choose the vegetarian options in the meal plans. You can also sprinkle a few pumpkin, sesame or sunflower seeds on your meals for essential fatty acids. I recommend you incorporate some B12 fortified foods into your diet. B12 is added to yeast extracts, soya milk and some breakfast cereals.

Q I've lost 9lb after two weeks on your Gi Jeans Kick-start Diet. Should I be concerned that I have lost so much or just pleased?

A This is perfectly normal and you should definitely be pleased, but it is also normal for the rate of weight loss to slow down in subsequent weeks. When we lose weight, a good proportion of what we lose initially is water. The carbohydrate we eat is stored in our muscles and liver in the form of a substance called glycogen. One gram of glycogen binds four grams of water to itself. When we go on a diet the body draws on its stores of glycogen (carbohydrate) for energy. Many slimmers have lost 9lb or more in the first two weeks of the diet and then gone on to lose 2lb or so each week after that.

Q I eat breakfast at 6.30am, which consists of two slices of wholemeal toast and tea. By 10.30am I'm getting really light-headed. How can I avoid this?

A It's a long time to go from 6.30am to 10.30am without food, so it makes sense to have a halfway snack between breakfast and lunch to keep your energy levels up. Try having a Power Snack (see page 138–9) or one of my Low Gi Nutrition Bars. Remember to include the calories in your daily total.

Q I'm following your Gi Jeans Diet but I don't drink alcohol. Can I have an extra treat each day?

A Yes, you can have an additional treat or snack each day worth 100 calories. While you are allowed one daily 100-calorie treat that is high in fat, make sure any extra ones you choose have a maximum of five per cent fat.

Q Is lemon juice a bonus on your Gi Jeans Diet? I have fresh lemon in tea and read somewhere that it helps when following the plan.

A Research shows that acidity can slow down the emptying of the stomach and therefore the rate of digestion of carbohydrate in food. This seems to occur when vinegar or lemon juice is added to a salad for instance. Lemon added to tea is unlikely to have the same effect but having lemon instead of milk reduces the calories. Remember, though, we need milk to supply our calcium needs, so try not to miss out by having milk with cereal or yogurt for dessert.

Q When following your diet, is there a limit to the amount of fat grams you can eat in one day?

A The total number of fat grams you eat in one day on my Gi Jeans Diet does not matter as long as the foods you choose are all five per cent or less fat and you stick to your calorie allowance. There are a few exceptions to the five per cent rule, such oily fish and some brands of wholegrain bread, because of their nutritional benefits, and of course your daily treat can be more than five per cent fat.

Q I have just completed your two-week Kick-start Diet and wondered if I could stay on this as I feel fine and don't get any hunger pangs.

A People over 60 with reduced calorie needs can stay on the Kick-start Diet for longer, as can anyone whose BMR gives them a calorie allowance of round 1300 a day. Other people should not follow it for longer than two weeks at a time as it could adversely affect the metabolism and cause it to slow down, making weight loss more difficult. You will lose weight successfully on the main diet plan.

Q Can tea or diet drinks count towards my water intake or does it have to be plain water – our tap water tastes awful?

A Water – still or sparkling – is the best choice. If you don't want to buy bottled water, I suggest you try a water filter jug, as it will significantly improve the taste of tap water and can be kept in the refrigerator. Tea – regular or flavoured – is also fine, as is up to three cups of coffee per day. Low-calorie soft drinks are acceptable, but avoid regular fizzy drinks as these contain lots of sugar, which won't help your weight-loss efforts.

Q I'm a vegetarian. Can I substitute Quorn for meat in the recipes?

A Yes, you can substitute Quorn for meat in any of the recipes. You can use the same quantity, although if this seems too large a portion, you might prefer to use less Quorn and have additional vegetables.

Q I have read somewhere that heating milk raises its Gi level. Is this true?

A Heating milk breaks down some of the milk protein, which makes it slightly easier to digest, but the effect on the Gi rating is minimal.

Q Do I have to stick to my three meals a day? I sometimes don't have time for lunch.

A Yes, you should stick to three main meals a day to keep your digestive system busy and your blood sugar levels up. Skipping meals will only make you crave the wrong type of foods. You could choose a prepacked sandwich or salad option or split lunch over a longer period of time if it suits you better.

Q Can I eat wholemeal bread instead of wholegrain bread on your Gi Jeans Diet?

A Wholemeal bread has a higher Gi rating than wholegrain bread, although it has more fibre than normal white or brown bread, both of which are high Gi. Adding baked beans will lower the Gi rating, though, so beans on wholemeal toast is also a good low-Gi option.

Q I don't like fruit and would rather have orange or apple juice. Is this OK?

A Fruit juice has a higher Gi than whole fruit and doesn't contain as much fibre. If you buy it readymade it can also include preservatives and added sugar, so check the ingredients on the nutrition panel. However, it's better to have fruit juice than no fruit at all. A small (150ml) glass has the same number of calories as a large orange. Choose juices that aren't made from concentrates as they taste better and have fewer additives. Better still, make yourself a smoothie. Do watch the amount you drink, though, as it's significantly higher in calories than water or sugar-free drinks.

Q Why do old potatoes have a higher Gi than new ones? Are they to be avoided completely on your Gi Jeans Diet?

A Potatoes that have been stored for some time have already begun to break down their starch. This means it takes less time for the starch to break down in the digestive system. However, you can reduce the Gi rating by serving an old jacket potato with a low-Gi topping such as baked beans. Alternatively, for a good low-Gi option, try baking sweet potatoes. With their orange colour and flesh they also contain the antioxidants beta carotene and vitamin C, are high in fibre and taste delicious.

Q I really love nuts and I read somewhere that nuts and seeds are recommended to help fight cancer, heart disease and high cholesterol. I know they are high in fat and I do want to lose weight. What should I do?

A The fat in nuts is mostly the unsaturated kind, particularly monounsaturated fat similar to that found in olive oil. Monounsaturated fat does not carry the same health risks as saturated fat, and can indeed protect against heart disease and help lower cholesterol. Recent research has shown that a 30-gram portion of nuts such as almonds per day will benefit health without causing weight gain. So providing you count them into your calorie allowance, nuts can be part of a healthy eating plan. You could also have some nuts as one of your treats but be very strict with the quantity. Avoid salted nuts as salt can have an adverse effect on blood pressure.

Q My husband has just treated us to a smoothie maker. The children love the drinks but I am concerned that they are high in calories and I am trying to lose weight. Can I have one occasionally?

A Smoothies can be made in a variety of ways. Some are made simply from fruit or fruit and water while others are made with yogurt, ice cream or even real cream! Also, some are sweetened with sugar or honey. Before making one for yourself, look at the recipe and work out the calories for your portion. Providing you count your calories into your allowance there is no reason why you shouldn't enjoy this healthy drink as a breakfast or part of your lunch. Try using an artificial sweetener or low-calorie granulated sugar to save a few extra calories.

Q I have recently given up buying ready meals because of all the bad reports about processed foods, too much sugar, salt, and so on. Now I am finding it really difficult to count the calories and watch the fat content of the meals that I am preparing and my weight has plateaued. Have you any tips?

A   There is no doubt that buying ready meals when you are
    dieting saves you time and it's helpful to have the calorie
content of each serving and the percentage of fat on the
label. As you rightly say, the sugar and salt content can be
excessive and this is not good for health. However,
manufacturers are now producing healthier options of
ready meals and the new signposting system on the front
of packs means it's easier to make the healthiest choices.
It's true, though, that preparing your own meals can be
cheaper and more nutritious. To measure the calorie
content of home-made meals you either have to weigh
your ingredients raw or after they are cooked. You need a
good calorie book or a set of my Nutri-Scales, which do all
the calculating for you. These very clever scales are
programmed with 500 different foods, you look up the
food you are about to eat in the chart provided, tap in the
code for that food and, once the food is on the scales,
they will tell you how many calories are in your portion.
You soon learn which foods to weigh raw (such as chicken
breast) or cooked (such as rice or pasta). Try to select
ingredients with five per cent or less fat (except oily fish)
and you will be able to make it work. You will soon get
into the swing of it and the reward will be seeing those
pounds and inches dropping away.

Q   I enjoy a glass of wine most evenings and I just have one
    glass and have always counted it as 100 calories. Because
we have small children I haven't been to the pub for years
but last week we went to our local with some friends. I
ordered a red wine and felt the barman was having a joke!
I could not believe that it was an actual pub measure of a

glass of wine – but it was. Please can you tell me how much wine I can have for my 100 calories?

A It's frightening isn't it! When you dine out, you pour out of the bottle and it is only in a pub or bar situation that you are actually served 'a glass'. The facts are that 150ml – and that's a small, old-style glass – of dry red or white wine is 100 calories. Some of those enormous but very stylish red wine glasses that we have now become used to can hold up to half a bottle and that's 250 calories!

Q I've read about the dangers of trans fats recently and understand that they are found in many manufactured foods. Is it advisable to avoid these foods completely when following your diet and will this help me to lose weight?

A Certainly, there is every reason to cut down on trans fats. They contain just as many calories as every other fat and are specifically linked to high cholesterol levels and heart disease in a similar way to saturated fat. Trans fats mostly occur in baked goods – everything from meat pies and pasties to biscuits and cakes. Anyone following my diets should really avoid these foods because of their high overall fat content. Choosing low-fat ready meals and, if you really can't live without it, a margarine specifically labelled as low in trans fats will also help minimise your intake of these harmful fats. The good news is that many food manufacturers in the UK are already working to decrease trans and saturated fat in their products, which will certainly help improve the nation's health.

Q I bought a sachet of soup and the label says it has six grams of fat per 100 grams of powder but that the 55-gram sachet contains only 0.2 grams of fat. Is it all right to have this on your diet or should I look for one with less than five grams of fat per 100 grams of powder?

A Good question. The confusion arises because the product is sold in a dehydrated state. When it is mixed with water, as per the packet instructions, it will 'dilute' the fat content to bring it right down to less than one per cent. The same applies to items such as custard powder and even porridge, all of which are fine on the diet and under five per cent fat when reconstituted.

Q I'm allergic to gluten and have to eat a gluten-free diet. Can I still follow your diet?

A The wide variety of choice in my eating plans means you can easily steer yourself away from foods that are not gluten-free. You can substitute rice or potatoes in place of pasta, buy gluten-free bread in place of regular wheat bread and create recipes using alternative thickening agents such as cornflour and arrowroot in place of normal flour. Also, check out www.coeliac.co.uk where you'll find lots of information and guidance as to which foods to choose and which to avoid.

Q I have been a Type 1 diabetic for 11 years and lost weight successfully before. However, I now I find it very hard to control sugars and lose weight and have put on over a stone. Will your Gi Jeans Diet work for me?

A A low-Gi diet is recommended for diabetics who want to lose weight and my Gi Jeans Diet is designed to give you sustained energy levels and keep blood sugar levels constant. Some diabetics are naturally a little nervous about restricting calories, so progress may be somewhat slower. But if you follow the diet and make sure you eat your Power Snacks at the correct times, there is no reason why you shouldn't succeed. However, I do recommend that anyone with Type 1 diabetes speak to their doctor or health professional before embarking on any weight-loss plan.

Q I would like to follow your diet, but I've struggled with diets in the past as I'm allergic to milk and dairy products. I can drink soya and rice milk and I like the Alpro soya yogurts, but I can't eat any cheese or cream.

A My diets are very adaptable and you can certainly have soya or rice milk in place of ordinary cow's milk and have soya yogurts in place of dairy ones. Just check the calories of the products to ensure that you keep within your daily allowance. Try also substituting beans and pulses in place of cheese and you should be able to adapt the diet without a problem.

Q I want to lose weight and get fitter but I am still breastfeeding my three-month-old baby. Can I still follow the diet? I have had all my postnatal checks and everything is fine so when can I start exercising?

A While you are still breastfeeding it is vital that you do not actually 'diet' but you can certainly eat very healthily and cut out high-fat snacks such as chocolate, sweets, biscuits, cakes and savoury snacks. Feed yourself a healthy, balanced diet of three meals a day and if you are really hungry between meals because of your milk production, eat healthy snacks such as a banana, pot of yogurt or a small bowl of cereal. Just try not to overeat. The good news is that you are breastfeeding and remember that the higher the quality of the food you eat the more nutritious will be your milk for your baby. You can take some easy exercise now that you have had your postnatal check-up but it is really important that you do not overdo it. Walking out with your baby is good for both of you and when you feel up to it, try some gentle aerobics at home or go to a Rosemary Conley class. All the instructors are qualified and trained to teach postnatal mums. The key is not to do too much too soon.

Q I am enjoying your diet but I struggle to drink the full 450ml (¾ pint) milk allowance. I don't like drinking milk on its own, so could I make it into a milk shake?

A Milk shake cordial is very high in sugar, so it will add unnecessary calories to your daily intake. It would be better to make a fresh fruit smoothie with strawberries or raspberries and flavour your milk this way. You can also use up some of your allowance with cereal for breakfast. Another alternative is to substitute 150ml (¼ pint) of milk with a pot of yogurt. The important thing is that you have sufficient calcium, which is needed for healthy bones and teeth, and the milk allowance is designed to supply most of your daily requirement.

Q I would like to follow your diet but will I lose weight off the tops of my legs? I stopped smoking a year ago and gained a stone in weight. I am 5ft 3in tall and weigh 10st 5lb. All the weight seems to have gone on the tops of my legs and they look huge and lumpy! I go to the gym three times a week and I walk for an hour a day too. Will I ever have slim legs again?

A It's tough when you are short because there is less area for the increased fat to be spread over! You are obviously pear-shaped and that is why you are storing your excess weight on your thighs. You need to lose the 14lb you have gained and when you do you will have much slimmer thighs, I promise. To minimise your fat deposits, eat a low-fat, calorie-controlled diet of around 1350 calories a day and keep up the regular exercise as this will really help. Your daily walk is a brilliant fat-burner for your legs as well as making you generally fitter. Try to combine some cardiovascular work in the gym with some body-toning strength work, particularly working your leg muscles to make them stronger. We burn fat in our muscles, so the stronger your leg muscles, the easier if will be for you to burn the fat from that area.

Q I am 60 years old and have osteoporosis and osteoarthritis in my neck and spine. I know your diet really works but I have been told by my physiotherapist that I should not exercise. Will I still be able to lose weight?

A It is such a shame that you are suffering in this way but the good news is that you can still lose weight, even without exercise. It just takes a little longer. Anyone over 60 needs to cut back the calories to lose weight as the body naturally uses fewer calories as we get older. Try to stick to around 1200–1300 calories a day and you will see those excess pounds reducing, albeit a little slowly.

Q I desperately want to lose some fat from my stomach and waist. Which exercise is best to help reshape this area?

A It sounds as if you are an apple shape, which means you naturally store fat around your tummy area. Following a low-Gi, calorie-controlled, low-fat diet, such as the one in this book, will help reduce your body fat, including the fat on your abdomen – and in trials we found that this is exactly the place people lost most inches from. But you need to exercise as well. Aerobic exercise such as walking, jogging or salsacise will burn fat, and the bigger and stronger your abdominal muscles are, the more effective the fat burning will be. So do some specific tummy and waist exercises (see page 300) to tone your muscles as well.

Q I am 5ft 5in tall and weigh 9st 3lb, so I'm not overweight but I do have lots of cellulite on my thighs and buttocks. If I follow your diet will I shift the cellulite or am I stuck with it for life?

A As you are carrying your fat stores on your hips and thighs you are obviously a pear shape. Eating a low-Gi, low-fat diet will definitely help you to stay lean but I think the key for you is aerobic exercise, which burns fat as well as making you fitter. My Gi Jeans Weight-loss Workout DVD contains two aerobic workouts. Brisk walking, running, aerobics to music and salsacise are also great fat-burners that really use the legs. Try to incorporate 20–30 minutes of activities like these that make you breathe more deeply and feel quite warm, on five days a week, and you'll be amazed at the difference it makes to your cellulite. Also drink plenty of water and massage in some body lotion after a bath or shower. The massaging action will help improve the circulation around your hips and thighs.

Q I had a hysterectomy five years ago which left me with a bikini line scar. I don't mind about that, but I have a bit of flesh that hangs over the scar. Is there any exercise I can do to help flatten it? I'm about a stone overweight.

A Scar tissue causes the skin to shrink slightly, particularly on a part of the body where we store fat, with the consequence that you are left with a little 'shelf'. But if you lost your excess weight I am sure your stomach would flatten out. Exercise-wise you need to do some fat-burning aerobic work to help you lose weight and burn off the fat deposited on your stomach. You should also try some tummy toning exercises (see page 300) to strengthen your abdominal muscles.

Q I have lost 3st on your diet and feel fantastic, but I need to lose another 10lb to reach my target. I find myself losing 1lb one week only to gain it the next. I'm getting really frustrated. Can you give any pointers?

A The problem is that when we have followed a weight-reducing diet for a while we get too confident and stop weighing our food and sneak a little extra here and there. But we honestly believe that we are sticking to the diet plan. For the next week write down every single item of food and drink you consume, as you eat and drink it, and weigh out your portions. Check that you are eating the exact meals listed in the menu plans. If you are making changes to the menus it could be you haven't accurately counted the calories. I am sure you will soon see where you are going wrong on the food front. Then start exercising a little more. Try getting up ten minutes earlier each day and go for a brisk walk before you have your shower or breakfast and you will be amazed at the results.

Q My daughter is 11 and wants to lose about 12lb. She is 5ft tall and weighs almost 9st. We all now eat a low-fat diet and I give her three smaller meals a day with two or three low-fat snacks to keep her going. However, I am worried by reports in the press of childhood obesity. What do you suggest?

A Your daughter is not obese and you are on the right track by introducing the whole family to low-fat eating. It would be wrong to isolate your daughter or to make too much of an issue of her size. She will grow into her weight if you can try to educate her away from high-fat snacks and towards greater physical activity, too. Also, as a family, try to become more active. Playing games in the garden, going for walks, going swimming or even working out to one of my DVDs or videos can be fun and extremely effective. It is good to take such a responsible attitude to healthy eating and activity and I suggest you avoid the word 'diet' and instead talk about a healthy way of eating.

Q My dad is 72 and he's been told to lose weight because he has high blood pressure. He lives on his own. Can he follow your diet and what's your advice?

A Start by asking your dad to write down everything he eats and drinks for a week. And I mean everything. Go through the list with him and point out any snacks he has between meals, how much alcohol he drinks and where there is a 'high fat' element to his diet, for instance pie and chips at his local café or pub, or cakes, biscuits and chocolate. Ask him to try eating fruit instead of high-fat snacks and to choose new potatoes instead of chips. If he enjoys quite a lot of alcohol, try to encourage him to cut back by a third initially. The main thing is to ensure he understands where the fat is in food so he can learn to avoid it. If he insists on having butter on his bread, steer him towards low-cholesterol spreads such as Benecol to help his heart condition.

Q I've lost 3st on your diet and I have maintained it for two years, having completely changed my attitude to food. Thank you. I can't tell you what a relief it is after years of paranoia about my weight. Then last week, I had a binge. It just came over me like a wave and I found myself prowling round looking for something naughty to eat. In the end, I remembered a box of unopened chocolates left over from Christmas and I ate the lot. I can't believe I did it. I dread going back to my old ways. What can I do?

A If it makes you feel any better, I did exactly the same thing a day after Mothering Sunday. My daughter brought me, amongst other lovely gifts, two luxury chocolates, which I ate immediately (she knows I couldn't be trusted with a whole box!) and a mini tub of Pringles, another of my favourites. I was 'prowling' for something naughty to eat and suddenly remembered the Pringles. I sat on the floor and ate them all, five at a time! What I ate wasn't that bad on reflection. What *was* bad was my attitude. I was deliberately looking for 'trouble' and that is so unlike how I am now. Food does not control me any more – except on that afternoon. I felt disgusted with myself but stopped myself doing more damage by going out and thinking about something completely different. I didn't allow myself to self-destruct. I then put the episode behind me. So don't panic. These moments will happen very occasionally. It's normal. But it does show how far we've moved forward from where we were.

Q I love bread but I have been told that it is bad to eat it after 3pm as it makes you retain water. Also I have been told to toast my bread as this will decrease the amount of calories. How much of this is true?

A You will be pleased to know that you can eat bread at any time. It does not cause water retention either. However, if you were to eat your bread spread or filled with high-salt butter or cheese, it may cause you to drink more but your wonderful digestive system will soon regulate and any extra fluid you have consumed will be passed in the normal way. On the bread vs toast question, in fact the toast will contain MORE calories than the bread if you take it on a strictly weight for weight comparison. The difference is the water content. When you toast the bread some of the water held in the bread will evaporate, making it weigh less. Water, of course, is calorie free but if you calculated your calories based on bread and then weighed it out as toast, you could be eating more calories than you think! The answer is to weigh your bread out as bread and then toast it if you want to.

Basal Metabolic Rate (BMR) Table

Women aged 18–29			Women aged 30–59			Women aged 60–74		
Body Weight			Body Weight			Body Weight		
Stones	Kilos	BMR	Stones	Kilos	BMR	Stones	Kilos	BMR
7	45	1147	7	45	1208	7	45	1048
7.5	48	1194	7.5	48	1233	7.5	48	1073
8	51	1241	8	51	1259	8	51	1099
8.5	54	1288	8.5	54	1285	8.5	54	1125
9	57	1335	9	57	1311	9	57	1151
9.5	60.5	1382	9.5	60.5	1337	9.5	60.5	1176
10	64	1430	10	64	1373	10	64	1202
10.5	67	1477	10.5	67	1389	10.5	67	1228
11	70	1524	11	70	1414	11	70	1254
11.5	73	1571	11.5	73	1440	11.5	73	1279
12	76	1618	12	76	1466	12	76	1305
12.5	80	1665	12.5	80	1492	12.5	80	1331

13	83	1712	13	83	1518	13	83	1357
13.5	86	1760	13.5	86	1544	13.5	86	1382
14	89	1807	14	89	1570	14	89	1408
14.5	92	1854	14.5	92	1595	14.5	92	1434
15	95.5	1901	15	95.5	1621	15	95.5	1460
15.5	99	1948	15.5	99	1647	15.5	99	1485
16	102	1995	16	102	1673	16	102	1511
16.5	105	2043	16.5	105	1699	16.5	105	1537
17	108	2090	17	108	1725	17	108	1563
17.5	111	2137	17.5	111	1751	17.5	111	1588
18	115	2184	18	115	1776	18	115	1614
18.5	118	2231	18.5	118	1802	18.5	118	1640
19	121	2278	19	121	1828	19	121	1666
19.5	124	2325	19.5	124	1854	19.5	124	1691
20	127	2373	20	127	1880	20	127	1717

Basal Metabolic Rate (BMR) Table

| Men aged 18–29 | | | Men aged 30–59 | | | Men aged 60–74 | | |
| Body Weight | | | Body Weight | | | Body Weight | | |
Stones	Kilos	BMR	Stones	Kilos	BMR	Stones	Kilos	BMR
7	45	1363	7	45	1384	7	45	1232
7.5	48	1411	7.5	48	1421	7.5	48	1270
8	51	1459	8	51	1457	8	51	1307
8.5	54	1507	8.5	54	1494	8.5	54	1345
9	57	1555	9	57	1530	9	57	1383
9.5	60.5	1602	9.5	60.5	1567	9.5	60.5	1421
10	64	1650	10	64	1603	10	64	1459
10.5	67	1698	10.5	67	1640	10.5	67	1497
11	70	1746	11	70	1676	11	70	1535
11.5	73	1794	11.5	73	1713	11.5	73	1573
12	76	1842	12	76	1749	12	76	1611
12.5	80	1890	12.5	80	1786	12.5	80	1649

13	83	1938	83	13	1822	83	13	1687
13.5	86	1986	86	13.5	1859	86	13.5	1725
14	89	2034	89	14	1895	89	14	1763
14.5	92	2082	92	14.5	1932	92	14.5	1801
15	95.5	2129	95.5	15	1968	95.5	15	1839
15.5	99	2177	99	15.5	2005	99	15.5	1877
16	102	2225	102	16	2041	102	16	1915
16.5	105	2273	105	16.5	2078	105	16.5	1953
17	108	2321	108	17	2114	108	17	1991
17.5	111	2369	111	17.5	2151	111	17.5	2028
18	115	2417	115	18	2187	115	18	2066
18.5	118	2465	118	18.5	2224	118	18.5	2104
19	121	2513	121	19	2260	121	19	2142
19.5	124	2561	124	19.5	2297	124	19.5	2180
20	127	2609	127	20	2333	127	20	2218

Weight-loss graph

Make up your own graph for each stone you lose, following the example below.

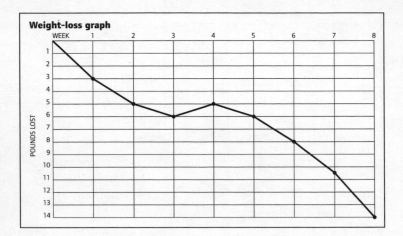

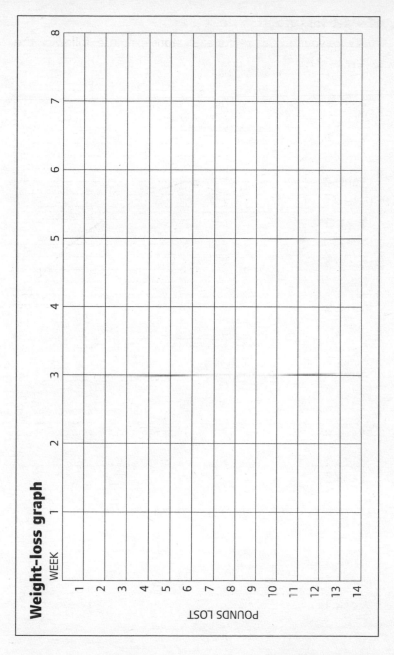

Weight-loss graph

WEEK

POUNDS LOST

	1	2	3	4	5	6	7	8
1								
2								
3								
4								
5								
6								
7								
8								
9								
10								
11								
12								
13								
14								

Weight-loss progress chart

	WEIGHT NOW	POUNDS/KG LOST	TOTAL LOSS TO DATE
Start day Date:			
Week 1 Date:			
Week 2 Date:			
Week 3 Date:			
Week 4 Date:			
Week 5 Date:			
Week 6 Date:			
Week 7 Date:			
Week 8 Date:			
Week 9 Date:			
Week 10 Date:			
Week 11 Date:			
Week 12 Date:			

	WEIGHT NOW	POUNDS/KG LOST	TOTAL LOSS TO DATE
Week 13 Date:			
Week 14 Date:			
Week 15 Date:			
Week 16 Date:			
Week 17 Date:			
Week 18 Date:			
Week 19 Date:			
Week 20 Date:			
Week 21 Date:			
Week 22 Date:			
Week 23 Date:			
Week 24 Date:			

How to measure yourself

Take the time to measure yourself once a week. It will provide the most encouraging proof of your progress, as sometimes we lose inches or centimetres when the scales are 'sticking'. Enter your measurements on the chart on page 358.

Widest measurement around the bust

Widest measurement around the upper arm

Smallest measurement around the waist

Widest measurement around the hips

Widest part should be the largest measurement in this area

Widest measurement around the thighs

Widest measurement above the knees

Measurement record chart

DATE	WEIGHT	BUST	WAIST	HIPS	WIDEST PART

TOP OF THIGHS		ABOVE KNEES		UPPER ARMS		TOTAL INCHES/CM LOST THIS WEEK	TOTAL INCHES/CM LOST TO DATE
L	R	L	R	L	R		

Exercise planner

	M	T	W	T	F	S	S
MORNING SESSION							
Aerobic workout 30 minutes	☐	☐	☐	☐	☐	☐	☐
Ultimate Gi Jeans Diet Workout							
Hips and thighs	☐	☐	☐	☐	☐	☐	☐
Tummy and waist	☐	☐	☐	☐	☐	☐	☐
LUNCHTIME SESSION							
Aerobic workout 30 minutes	☐	☐	☐	☐	☐	☐	☐
Ultimate Gi Jeans Diet Workout							
Hips and thighs	☐	☐	☐	☐	☐	☐	☐
Tummy and waist	☐	☐	☐	☐	☐	☐	☐
AFTERNOON/ EVENING SESSION							
Aerobic workout 30 minutes	☐	☐	☐	☐	☐	☐	☐
Ultimate Gi Jeans Diet Workout							
Hips and thighs	☐	☐	☐	☐	☐	☐	☐
Tummy and waist	☐	☐	☐	☐	☐	☐	☐

Steps per day record chart

	DATE	TARGET STEPS	ACTUAL STEPS
Day 1			
Day 2			
Day 3			
Day 4			
Day 5			
Day 6			
Day 7			
Day 8			
Day 9			
Day 10			
Day 11			
Day 12			
Day 13			
Day 14			
Day 15			
Day 16			
Day 17			
Day 18			
Day 19			
Day 20			
Day 21			
Day 22			
Day 23			
Day 24			
Day 25			
Day 26			
Day 27			
Day 28			

Index of recipes

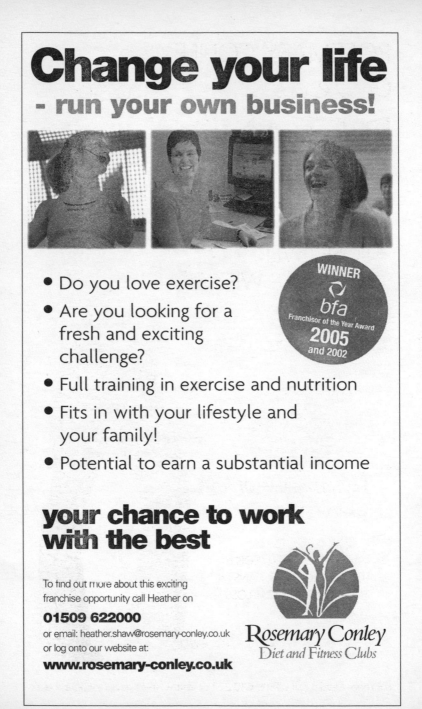

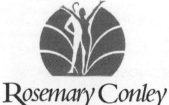

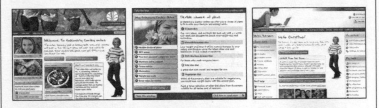

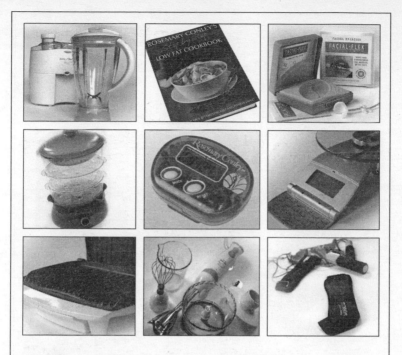

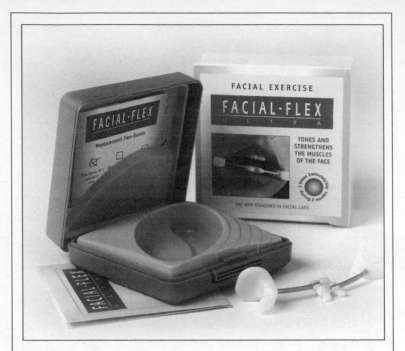
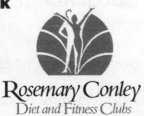

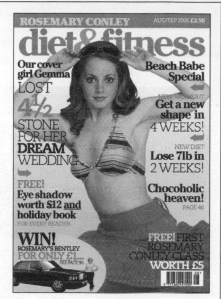

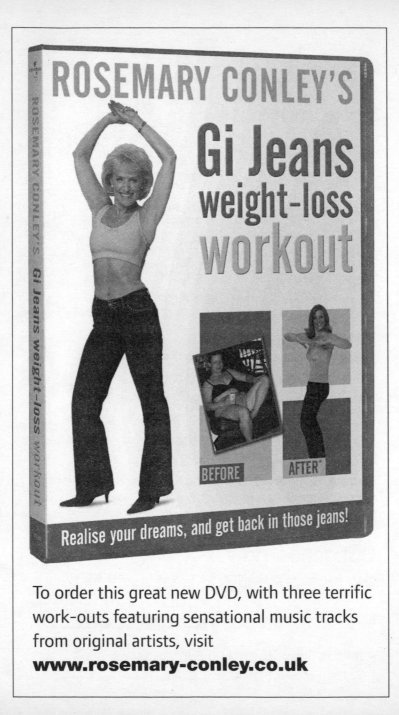